056712

HV 5808 .B55

Blum, Richard H.

Drug education

DATE DUE		
0 3 APR 1999		
1 3 DEC 2001		
DEC 1 9 2003		

Mill Woods

© THE BAKER & TAYLOR CO.

Drug Education: Results and Recommendations

Drug Education: Results and Recommendations

Richard H. Blum
Stanford University
with
Eva Blum and
Emily Garfield

Lexington Books
D.C. Heath and Company
Lexington, Massachusetts
Toronto

Library of Congress Cataloging in Publication Data

Main entry under title:
   Drug education.

   Bibliography: p.
   1. Drug abuse—Study and teaching—United States. I. Blum, Richard H.
HV5808.D786   362.2'9'071073   75-45821
ISBN 0-669-00575-4

Published simultaneously in Canada.

Printed in the United States of America.

International Standard Book Number: 0-669-00575-4

Library of Congress Catalog Card Number: 75-45821

Contents

List of Figures   ix

List of Tables   xi

Acknowledgments   xiii

Chapter 1   Introduction   1

Chapter 2   Children's Drug Use and its Educational Implications   9

Drug Findings: Outcomes as Interaction Effects   9

Chapter 3   Speaking of Education: Approaches   25

Process Education   34
Character Education?   42
The Range of Strategies   44
Resource Commentaries   46

Chapter 4   The Evaluation of Drug Education   47

A Clinical Evaluation   49
Educational Impact   50
A Question about Measurement   58

Chapter 5   The Research Design and the Drug Use Test: What We Did   63

Our Measures   65
Obtaining Other Information: School Records   66
Family Evaluation   66
Clinical Observations   66
Validity and Reliability of Self-Reports   67
Assignment   67
Substudies on Other Influences within the Educational Experience   67
Consumer Satisfaction and Recommendations   68
Curriculum   68
The Self-Report of Drug Use   68
Our Own Versus Other Estimates of Use   69

The High School Reliability Study   70
Our Drug Use Classification Scheme   71
Different Kinds of Tests: Visual versus
    Written   74
Comparing Two Different Questionnaire Forms   74
Measuring Declining Use   75
Summary   75

Chapter 6   **Drug Use and the Impact of Drug Education**   77

Drug Use   77
The Impact of Drug Education   85
Summary   98

Chapter 7   **Predicting Stability and Change**   99

School Characteristics   99
The Influence of Family Characteristics   114
Summary   120

Chapter 8   **Inhalant Users: A Special Case**   125

Inhalant Use   125
Educational Experience   130
Characteristics Associated with Inhalant
    Use   131
Comment and Summary   131

Chapter 9   **Consumer Evaluations**   133

Students   133
Educator Reactions   139
Parents   140
Summary   140

Chapter 10   **The Educational Climate**   143

Introduction   143
Educational Climate in Four Schools   144
The Student Backgrounds   149

Chapter 11   **Parental Influence and Children's Responses**   151

Introduction   151
Do Parents Have a Teaching Role?   152
What Students Hear   155
Other Actions   158

Chapter 12	**Reactions in the Classroom**	161
	Student Characteristics	161
	Summing Up Chapters 10, 11, and 12	166
Chapter 13	**Final Comment and Recommendations**	169
	Overview	169
	Strategy: Policy Options for School Intervention	175
	References	191
	Index	203
	About the Authors	219

List of Figures

6-1a   Estimated Prevalence Levels for Abstainers and Sanctioned Usage (Patterns 1, 2, and 3)   78

6-1b   Estimated Prevalence Levels for Marijuana Usage (Patterns 4 and 5)   79

6-1c   Estimated Prevalence Levels for Amphetamine, Barbiturate, and Psychedelic Usage (Patterns 6 and 7)   80

6-1d   Estimated Prevalence Levels for Heroin and Cocaine Usage (Patterns 8 and 9)   81

6-2   Drug Level Stability among Cohorts   84

6-3a   Estimated Percentage of Cohorts that Remain Stable within Drug Pattern (2) over a Two-year Period, All Students Starting from Pattern (2)   89

6-3b   Estimated Percentage of Nonstable Cohorts Reporting Extreme Pattern Change (10% Criterion) over a Two-year Period, All Students Starting from Pattern (2)   90

6-4a   Estimated Percentage Disadvantage of the Didactic (Y) and Process (Z) Modes over the Control (X) Based on the Criterion of Maintaining Stability   92

6-4b   Estimated Percentage Advantage of the Didactic (Y) and Process (Z) Modes over the Control (X) Based on the Criterion of Conditional Extremes   93

7-1   Accuracy of Prediction of Stable or Extreme Drug Use Patterns   112

8-1   Inhalant Use among Cohorts   126

8-2   Estimated Prevalence of Inhalant Use by
       Grade, Utilizing Subsample Written Test
       and Margin Calculated on Inconsistency
       Rates   128

List of Tables

5-1	Composition of the Research Sample	65
7-1	Sources for Student Characteristics	100
13-1	Drug Education Strategies	178

Acknowledgments

The research reported here was supported by Research Grant #DA 00097 (formerly MH #20220), National Institute for Drug Abuse. Technical support from the International Research Group on Drug Legislation and Programs (Geneva) and of the Drug Abuse Council (Washington, D.C.) is appreciated. The assistance rendered by the staff of NIMH and NIDA was invaluable, in particular Doctors Louise Richards, Robert Peterson, Richard Myrick, and Eleanor Carroll. In addition, we are indebted to the school district administrators and the teachers, pupils, and parents of our participant schools in San Mateo County. Exceptional aid was provided by Lillian Blackford, Nelson Burdett, Richard Genasci, Allen Gruman, Edith Hurley, Richard Irizary, Marilyn Kelly, J. Russell Kent, Ralph Paradise, Claudia Sampson, Roger Seccombe, and Anthony Steiner.

We also wish to acknowledge the considerable help rendered by the following: Ruth Arcand, Linda Barnett, Margery Bentley, Mary Fauvre, Virginia Fisher, Helen Foerster, William Hancock, Etta Hansen, Kenneth Helms, Eileen Hodge, Margaret Huntsberger, Judy Johnstone, Donald Jones, Therese Jordan, Peggy Joseph, Mary Klein, Iris Kriegler, John Magistad, Janet Pagen, Florence Schwartz, Ann Thomson, Cheryl Weeks, Edith Wieser, Kathryn Winterbotham, and Lawrence Wonderling.

Drug Education: Results
and Recommendations

1 Introduction

This book is about drug education. It tells of a four-year study of the effects of drug education and offers strategies for educators to apply in their communities. Our purpose is to provide information useful to teachers and administrators, to school counseling and health personnel, and to social scientists, community leaders, and parents who are concerned about children's drug use and the impact of education on that use. Our premises are that drug education is and will continue to be important and that drug education can be a strong influence on children's drug conduct. The concept of choosing strategies to fit various conditions arises from the fact of that influence, because it can be negative as well as positive, and because under some conditions there is expense without any influence at all.

There are a number of reasons why drug education deserves careful consideration, evaluation, and sophistication in its application. Consider the following:

1. By the time they leave high school the majority of American youngsters will be regular users of several psychoactive drugs and will have experimented with others, including illicit substances.

2. An important minority of youngsters, by the time they leave high school, will have suffered one or more ill effects in association with their drug use, as, for example, physical distress or accident.

3. Most parents are concerned about the moral and health aspects of drug use and many are concerned lest their own children develop either disapproved or actually self-endangering drug use habits.

4. Most parents want the schools to help guide their youngsters toward safe and approved lives, including drug use practices. Parents see the schools as a necessary complement to their own child rearing efforts, the schools providing information and "moral support" to that family-based effort.

5. Teachers and school administrators, along with other community leaders, are concerned about children's drug conduct. Their concerns arise not only on moral grounds but also because school personnel often directly observe acute drug effects which bear directly on teaching and learning, as in the case of the excited or sedated child, or because teachers are aware of the correlation between poor school performance, delinquency, and drug use.

6. School personnel are involved in drug concerns upon which drug education has a bearing. Children ask drug-related questions about which teachers want to be informed so that the adequacy of the teacher's own

1

education is pertinent. Teachers as human beings may also use psychoactive drugs, be these alcohol, tobacco, aspirin, or coffee; sedatives or stimulants with or without prescription; or, for that matter, marijuana. As consumers they want safely to guide themselves as well as their classroom charges.

7. Although the psychoactive drugs have been of primary public concern—those chemicals which affect states of mind, moods, sensory and thought processes, or biological cycles of sleep and wakefulness—there is increasing awareness that the child, as a growing consumer, will be using many other chemicals in his lifetime. Be these prescription or over-the-counter medications, industrial and household materials, or other compounds, there is a need for the consumer to be informed. Information ranges from matters of safety and efficacy to indications for use, costs, and environmental effects. Drug education increasingly occurs in the context of education for health care and for being a wise consumer.

8. Drug education exists. It is costly, on the order of several hundred million dollars per year over the nation, as measured in terms of teacher salaries, school overhead, and materials.

9. Drug education can have an impact that is negative, for, under some conditions, it increases favorable attitudes toward and an actual increase in the use of some psychoactive drugs, including illicit substances some of which contain high risks.

10. Drug education symbolizes the burden placed on the schools to prepare children, not simply to have skills and facts at their disposal, but to hold a given set of values and attitudes that are deemed to be in the service of their own health and adjustment and that conform to the community's view of propriety.

11. Drug education is one of the few interventions which society can employ which is both preventive and, on a per capita basis, cheap. Along with the family, the school is the only institution with a formative influence over children prior to the years when drugs become available to them and self-administered use begins. Education, unlike arrest or treatment, can be applied before either bad habits or bad outcomes have arisen.

In addition to these current reasons, one can expect increasing attention to drug education in the future if current trends continue. One of these trends is the expansion of self-administered drug use by children, and another is the availability of new compounds to youngsters. Political-economic forces also play a role. Insofar as school systems see drug education as a lever by which to claim more staff, power, and money, or legislators see it as a response to pressures to decentralize the Federal role and increase community work, then expansionist pressures will be felt. It will be well under such circumstances to know what to do, and to know what to do one had best be clear about terms as well as impact.

Drug education usually claims to help "prevent drug abuse." What does this mean? The term "drug abuse" is a semantic quagmire—meanings vary with the speaker and the context of the moment. It can refer to conduct which is illegal, unhealthy, immoral, simply unusual, or which symbolizes people or life styles which are disapproved. It is well to be as specific as possible in setting forth the kinds of drugs, users, settings, associated conduct and outcomes, and the standards for judgment under discussion.

What is meant by "drug education" may by no means always be evident either. Beyond the implication that there is an intention to do something about "drug abuse," what actually is practiced varies broadly. One has to say what the content of that effort is, where it takes place, what kinds of students are involved, what the teachers really do, what the objectives are, what the student perceives, and how he or she actually responds. The design and content of our study arose from our assumptions about the nature of children's drug use development and of the hazards which might arise, and from our notions of our civic and professional obligations to parents and teachers, to the communities in which we worked, to our scientific colleagues, and to the children themselves. Before we ventured into the schools we drew up a protocol describing our intentions, our definitions, and what our operating rules would be. That protocol is available upon request.

There will be continuing local and national investigations and discussions about drug education. These are necessary for the clarification of goals and for identifying the methods best suited to given student populations. That clarification requires that one be aware of personal and cultural values and also have an understanding of the many different kinds of drug use. As one considers educational objectives, one must ask: What assumptions and priorities are held? Is the aim to encourage conventionality and discourage unusual drug conduct? Is one interested in striving for the moral-religious goal of total abstinence from pleasure-giving substances? Is one primarily interested in health and therefore desirous of reducing only those drug use activities that can be shown empirically to be associated with illnesses like lung cancer (tobacco), cirrhosis of the liver (alcohol), abscesses, heart disease, and hepatitis (associated with nonsterile needles), liver damage (inhalants such as glue), psychotic episodes (amphetamines, LSD), or coma and death (barbiturate, opiate, and alcohol overdoses)? If health is the major concern does one also want to move beyond the prevention of possible damages to an interest in the benefits that drugs may offer? There is, for example, medical literature showing the benefits of wine; there are strong data showing how amphetamines improve fatigue-retarded performance; it is common knowledge that sedatives induce sleep and opiates relieve pain; and there are indications that marijuana will be found to have medical utility.

Alternatively, the educator may be interested in fostering life styles rather than stressing particular acute specific drug effects. In that instance, both the pharmacology of drug dependence and the personal preoccupation and social life centering on drugs which may constitute "addiction," might predominate in the preventive emphasis. Or is one concerned primarily about interpersonal behavior, for example, by having students avoid the drug-related aggressiveness or impulsiveness which can arise from some drug use? Accident prevention may also be an objective, as may be the illumination of the relationship between kinds of drugs, youngsters, and delinquency. There are those additional objectives which accompany consumer education or the teaching of the wise utilization of medicines other than psychoactive drugs during health care. Household safety with chemicals can be a related subject.

There are other powerful objectives which are arguably pertinent to any drug education which is concerned with that youthful drug use which arises from other than normal curiosity, sociability, recreation, or conventionality. Although catalogues of motives can be untrustworthy, and research findings on the preconditions for unusual, disapproved, or dangerous drug use are sometimes debated, it is safe to say that the drug-using youngsters who are most likely to get in repeated trouble will be different than normal youngsters: often they will come from defective families, will have personalities characterized as deficient or poorly adjusted, and will live in social environments that are not wholesome. It is no wonder that those concerned with deviant drug users become interested in mental health programs; argue for more affectionate, disciplined, informed, and attentive child rearing in the home; seek to provide constructive alternatives to the escapist, hedonistic, or unsafe self-medicating drug use of such youngsters; strive to develop character education as such; and campaign for alternative and restorative social environments which are not criminogenic or educationally adverse.

Drug education can be a lever by which advocates try to change schooling itself. Insofar as children may be seen to suffer disaffections which the ordinary school does not correct and which are said to be part of the genesis of extreme drug use, then the school more than the child can be the target for action. One finds these arguments in connection with those children who are bored in school, those who perform badly, those who are insensitively handled by school personnel, those who find school irrelevant to their life situations and goals, those who rebel against the values inherent in most American schools, and those who are considered, by some idealogues, as either oppressed or discarded by current education. Environmentalists that attribute extreme drug use to existing sociopolitical institutions may even seek to use "drug abuse prevention" as the wedge for major social reforms beyond the schoolgrounds.

These illustrative objectives show the array of intentions which drug education may have, many of which are not mutually exclusive, and point up the connection between drug education and one's own view of the world. What is good and bad, what accounts for unusual conduct, where does responsibility lie, and what methods for either prevention or change are desirable? Most educators will hold normal world views, including their evaluations of children's drug use and its multiple forms, origins, and consequences. Yet one must identify and reflect upon one's own beliefs and subject them to the test of present knowledge if one is to select an objective and rational strategy for drug education from among those available.

At the very least the responsible choice of educational strategies requires that the teacher and school administrator be informed about children's drug use and what it can signify. It means that there must be sensitivity to the variety of different instructional audiences. This is evident enough when one considers that 2nd graders will require different teaching than 8th graders, or as one examines the different patterns of drug use among children and their separate risks of differing outcomes. The concept of different levels of abilities and needs is hardly new to educators, any more than is their awareness of the value of fitting the teaching to the child. It is simply that this awareness must be extended to drug education, acknowledging that here—where the goal usually involves some kind of personal and social behavior—things are more complex. Children will probably respond differently to drug education depending not only on their age and classroom aptitudes, but also on their personalities, the kinds of drug experiences they have had, the subcultural, socioeconomic, and peer groups of which they are members, and their parents' moral views. Some of these same factors determine drug risks as well, that is, they are components in patterns of conduct which predict that child A has a greater chance of trying barbiturates than child B, or that teenager C has a greater risk of having alcohol problems than teenager D.

Suppose that we know that one youngster, aged fourteen, because of his personal and social characteristics has a greater likelihood of becoming a heroin user and later an addict than does his classmate. Preventive measures are limited, for within the school setting one is quite restricted in terms of the educational effort that can be mounted. It is generally considered unwise to single out children simply on the basis of their risk of some unhappy outcome, for to label a child in advance as a potential problem could possibly create damage that would not have occurred otherwise. It can also be an unjust interference in his life. Teachers and educational policy makers are aware, of course, of these labeling problems. They are also aware that within a drug educational curriculum there is precious little opportunity to diversify and individualize efforts. The exception may be opportunity for referral to some mental health, counseling, or other consulting person.

The concepts of probability are understood in most educational efforts. We know that some children will learn history while others will not. Some will learn to brush their teeth but nevertheless will develop dental caries. In the case of drug education, some may learn facts but will not change their already existing drug use conduct; others may become involved in classroom discussions and decide on that basis to forego barbiturates, but will nevertheless take up smoking cigarettes. Even when one has scientifically up-to-date information at hand about children's characteristics as linked to one or another drug-using career, it is still a matter of estimates. For example, it may happen that 70 percent of the children with pattern A use marijuana, but only 12 percent will go on to use LSD, and of these 12 percent, only a very few will suffer any emotional or thinking disorder associated with the LSD use. Since the uncertainty devils the scientist, the educational policy maker, and the teacher, uncertainty will also probably characterize the materials communicated to students. They must share with us our unsureness about those who will suffer some adverse reaction or undesirable result.

The best general estimate using existing data is that most children will use their drugs fairly safely, or even if some acute reaction does occur, will survive in spite of sickness or trouble. A few will die as youngsters, and more will die as adults, in association with drug-related diseases, reactions, or accidents. The other side of this chancy coin of adversity is that many individuals will enjoy their drug use. Why not? After all, many people appreciate the benefits of psychoactive drugs to help sleep, relax, be alert, diet, or fight "tension" headaches. Most adults enjoy the social facilitation and euphoria of alcohol, the reassurance of cigarettes, or the stimulation of coffee. Coffee or tobacco habitués know the relief of the distress of "withdrawal" if one has not had one's drug recently enough. Indeed, as new teachers are recruited from the ranks of recent college graduates, many among them have tried marijuana and found it enjoyable. Some teachers will have tried other drugs as well and found these an interesting experience.

These facts can present teachers with problems in their goal setting for drug education. One possible difficulty is that the teacher will feel uneasy telling the truth, fearing to acknowledge that human beings are almost universally drug-using animals who derive various satisfactions or reliefs from psychoactive drugs. The teacher may worry that objective information will not discourage students from engaging in disapproved drug conduct, or will be misinterpreted by parents and administrators who, on hearing a child's report, might conclude that the conscientious teacher is too liberal. A second possible problem is that teachers' own drug use habits—ranging from abstinence to serious alcoholism—may color the presentation, warping the facts to conform to the teacher's personal bias. In either of the above problem instances, drug education—insofar as it seeks to be soundly informative or to engage in objective discussions with children—may stand accused of distortions. Yet many communications on important personal and social affairs reflect personal feelings, cultural values, and prevailing political themes. Drug education should not expect to bear a purer truth than other teachings conveyed by caring humans in typical school environments. Drug education need not be more biased simply because it is such a sensitive, personal, and important subject. The personal commitment of the educator, therefore, should be to remain as objective as possible, including the objective appraisal of one's own beliefs, of how society responds to various drugs and their users, and of how users and nonusers feel about drug habits.

The decision of the educator as to what he or she seeks to accomplish and how best to go about it requires yet one more set of data: knowledge of the actual impact of drug education materials and methods available to the educator. That knowledge can come only through evaluation of what happens to children as a consequence of their exposure to a given educational program.

Some sociological cynics, looking at the inconsequential outcomes of early educational efforts, say that the success of drug education is in its failure. One foreign scholar commented that drug education is the opiate of American legislators. There is merit in such criticism insofar as drug education advocates have been exploiting the anxieties of citizens to offer panaceas, to pad budgets, or to undermine sound teaching by catering to mindless fashion or nonsensical pedagogical theory. Such criticism is warranted whenever an idea or program is offered without reflection or critical examination. On the other hand such criticism can overlook functions which are not identified in outcome statistics, as for example, the "doing something" which humans find so necessary when they are in trouble or the "moral support" which parents tell us they want from the schools. Drug education performs those functions. The criticism also overlooks the disadvantages of efficiency. If any institution under governmental control were to become adept at molding beliefs and character, effectively programming the people who emerge from such "processing," what would be the threats to diversity and freedom? Certainly as a society we are now paying dearly for the failure of families to raise children who are as socially responsible as they are free, but the alternative of schools that are indeed capable of efficiently homogenizing humans is disturbing.

The most important reply to the denunciation of success because of failure is the converse: drug education's success can be in its actual impact. We have found that particular methods applied at certain grade levels do work. Drug education is effective when effectiveness is measured by a less-than-expected expansion of use over a several-year period into more unusual, more disapproved substances, what some people call the "hard" drugs: amphetamines, barbiturates, opiates, cocaine, and hallucinogens. Education is effective in these same conditions when it is measured by student satisfaction. School boards and school administrators also approve. But drug education as we practiced and tested it has another impact, the "negative" impact of increasing the movement into and rate of use of the conventional psychoactive drugs: alcohol, tobacco, and marijuana. The effects vary from high to low depending upon the grade level of students and depending upon the educational method applied.

These findings lead to the concept of educational strategies. The selection of the "best-fit" approach depends upon community drug use levels and exposure, the existence of visible cases of ill effects or delinquency, the commitment to broad versus narrow "drug abuse prevention" objectives, and the age at which children in a school are showing a critical expansion of their drug interests and experimentation.

In brief, the strategy avoids classroom drug education pertaining to "drugs of abuse" in communities where levels of use of all drugs are low, where abstinence is common, and where there is no immediate outlook for increased exposure. The other extreme occurs in individual schools where levels of self-administered psychoactive drug use are high, where there are a significant number of "bad outcomes," where the expectation is that without intervention there will be an expansion of use into more unusual substances, and when there is a community commitment to action. There the strategy recommended is (1) regular community monitoring of childrens' drug use levels keyed to age; (2) drug education applied preventively at those age levels where children are otherwise expected to begin to expand their use; (3) use of objective and evaluated teaching materials, as for example, the experimental curriculum which we developed; and (4) the simultaneous utilization of referrals to community agencies and the exercise by the school of strong efforts to control any and all illicit drug use on its premises, including tobacco. In between and supplemental to these major strategic alternatives there are others. Further discussion of strategies appears in the final chapter.

The rationale for these recommendations and the selection of strategic options by individual schools arises from the research on drug education which our group at Stanford has conducted. That work includes a series of studies on youthful drug use extending back to 1962. In addition, many research and demonstration efforts by others have been an important influence on our thinking, as has been our personal experience.

Basic is the conviction that one part of policy must rest on what drug education achieves as measured by children's drug use. That knowledge should not be the sole factor in policy making, for while there is a correlation between levels of use and hazardous outcomes, the relationship is complex and by no means unvarying. Furthermore, empiricism is not a complete guide; practical, political, and ideological factors will influence what school systems do. But findings from research must play a part in educational policy, and insofar as the objectives include real changes in children's drug use, then the educational effort must be tested through evaluation using scientifically adequate methods.[a] Without evaluation the taxpayer does not know whether he is getting his money's worth for his educational dollar. It is therefore the obligation of administrators and teachers to make their "drug abuse prevention" objectives clear, to set up standards by which to test whether the goals have been achieved, and to experiment with different teaching methods—or the manipulation of school environments—to see whether one can do better than before. In each instance one must compare the costs and benefits. These are steps in rational decision making about drug education. It is the same kind of rationality which teachers hope to instill in the decision making of youth. Drug education can be the model for such rationality, both in youngsters and in school policy. As such it can provide an opportunity for youngsters to live wiser lives, and to demonstrate to an increasingly skeptical public that educators are clear headed, effective, cost conscious, and genuinely caring professionals and public servants.

---

[a]We shall not pursue the argument in favor of objective evaluation further here. For anyone interested in an account of the benefits—and the pitfalls—of evaluation research, along with information on how to design and manage such studies, we recommend reading *Accountability in Drug Education*. That monograph, edited by Abrams, Garfield, and Swisher, is published by the Drug Abuse Council, 1828 L Street N.W., Washington, D.C. 20036.

2 Children's Drug Use and Its Educational Implications

In this chapter we shall draw on some of the scientific work done to date, generalizing from it so as to present a view of some of the major social correlates of children's drug use. We shall also consider the implications of that knowledge for the educational enterprise. This chapter does not report on the findings of our own drug education research. That report begins with Chapter 5.

There has been much research since the early 1960s bearing on children's and young people's drug use. The findings, when put together, yield a fairly complete picture of what children use which drugs in what ways. Considerable attention has been paid not only to these career, developmental, etiological, and epidemiological features, but to examining how a drug, a person, and a setting interact to yield a particular reaction or outcome. There has also been sociological inquiry into societal reactions, as, for example, how others view a drug-using person and what the consequences are. The scientific work done ranges from the disciplines of biochemistry and genetics to studies of social policy. The findings of interest to the drug educator or the drug scientist, therefore, can range from a knowledge of how a particular nerve cell receptor site fits, like a lock for a key, into the molecule of heroin which binds to it, to a knowledge of how heroin use is taught via a friendship network by older to younger youths.

Drug Findings: Outcomes As Interaction Effects

One of the most helpful contributions of research to the development of educational policy lies in the recognition that much of what once were considered to be specific pharmacological effects (i.e., biochemical reactions) are really interaction effects in which psychological and social factors play a role together with pharmacological ones. It has been demonstrated (Becker, 1963) that people not only learn to use drugs, but they learn to expect and interpret their reactions in different ways depending upon how those around them exercise their influence. Within the ordinary dosage range for psychoactive drugs there is also a range of variability which can occur in terms of what people feel or how they act. Over the long term there are a variety of courses open to people in the styles of their drug use and the social careers that emerge. What determines these reactions and careers is a complex mix of personal, environmental, and biochemical events, and thus one cannot understand how humans

9

come to use or to react to particular drugs without knowing about their expectations, motives, personality adjustments, life values, and the like. One certainly needs to know about pharmacology if the picture is to be drawn completely, but for understanding events at the level of intervention represented by the school itself when it practices drug education, the corresponding levels of social and psychological events are more pertinent.

The psychosocial factors that influence drug use and outcomes—whether immediate reactions or long-term life styles—are derived not only from personality features, but also from family, peers, setting, and society itself. In conducting drug education, the school and the teacher are themselves seeking to be such influences on drug use patterns. One fact pertaining to the teaching influence is that predispositions to use or avoid use are general as well as drug specific in nature. There is an attitudinal set which can range from intense and general disapproval of the self-administered social or private use of any drug to strong advocacy of the use of almost any drug. Associated with these attitudinal positions are found positive correlations in the use or nonuse of a variety of substances. If, for example, a youngster does not drink or smoke he is likely to disapprove of this conduct in himself and others, and will not be willing to try other drugs, such as street barbiturates or marijuana. On the other hand, if one knows that a high school student smokes cigarettes heavily, then one can make a good guess that he is also likely to use alcohol and, if illicit drugs are available in his neighborhood or school, he is more of a candidate for experimentation and perhaps regular use than is a nonsmoker. Thus, if one examines drug use, one will see that the typical patterns are of multiple use, with the patterns differentiated by intensity of use and by the extent to which the more disapproved substances are employed. One can also rely on such correlations to identify stages in use (Kandel, 1975; Jessor and Jessor, 1974; Goldstein, 1975).

One can make a scale, based on the prevalence of use in a community, whereby drugs are ranked from the most commonly to the least commonly used outside of medical practice. This scale corresponds roughly to the levels of social approval or fear of a drug. In most United States cities alcohol and tobacco are the substances most commonly used by adults and by youngsters, cannabis (marijuana) ranks second for young people, amphetamines and barbiturates (not prescribed) are less often used, and the opiates are least used. For a youngster already using at any one of these levels, one can estimate that since he has already employed the more common drugs as compared with people not yet at his place on the scale, he is much more likely than less-experienced youngsters to try an even less approved drug; that is, one only rarely used in the community.

There are personal, social, and residential characteristics which assist one in predicting which young people will be ready to move up the scale to use a less-common substance. These same features will generally be correlated with intensity of use. For a given drug, whether it is alcohol or LSD, the people who have more of the traits generally associated with the use of that drug—or with a predilection to use any psychoactive substance—are more likely to use the drug more often and in larger amounts. Increase in use and dosage is ordinarily associated with an increased risk of adverse outcomes in association with the drug, as, for example, centering one's life on drugs so as to be classified as an addict, having illnesses arise from the drug, suffering arrest or social difficulty, and the like. These are probabilities that can be used best when predicting for groups of people; the best prediction for an individual tends to be the same prediction that would be made for the majority of persons with his or her same characteristics.

In addition to these general statements, which apply across the board for the social or private use of all psychoactive drugs available in a community, there are particular predictors linked to drug preferences or levels of use. For example, if one becomes a member of a social group in which one substance is fashionable, then the risk of learning to use it is much higher. In our study we found very high use of inhalants (gasoline, glue, paint thinner, etc.) among the girls in one class in one school. As these girls were promoted, their inhalant use tapered off, possibly because of reassignment to different classes and a change in close peer relationships. But growth as such also makes a difference: inhaling is reduced as users grow older. Other studies have found that heroin use is higher in some poor neighborhoods than in others; for example, heroin use depends on the mix of neighborhood ethnic groups as well as within-family factors such as the absence of a father, and on peer features such as the presence of a nearby friendship group of heroin-using peers. Predisposing to one form of early alcoholism is the cultural pattern—France is a good example—whereby parents who view the water as unsafe give their children wine instead. Over the years children develop a pharmacological dependency on the alcohol, but may never realize it until some situation arises whereby they do not get to drink their ordinary wine ration and then begin to suffer withdrawal or the "abstinence syndrome," as, for example, delirium tremens.

Other sets of predisposing factors may be found in the immediate family. If parents teach their children to use substances such as wine, cigarettes, marijuana, or heroin, the children readily become users. There is a strong relationship between what parents do and believe and what children come to do and believe. In our own research with families (Blum and Associates, 1972a) we found that quite successful prediction of the level and risk of teenagers' drug use could be based on knowledge of parental religion (the more religious, the less use), parental liberalism (the more liberal, the more use), family closeness (the closer, the less use), and parental drug use (the more parental use, the more child use, including prescription as well as recreational drugs). When it came to predicting not simply use or nonuse, but what we considered the risk of a bad outcome (illness, arrest, etc.), these same factors still held, but added to them were socially disruptive and psychopathological features. That is, when the families were not only irreligious, liberal, and drug using but were also ones where there was lack of love and humor, a parental inability to exercise care and discipline, or a great deal of parental anger, selfishness, or emotional instability, then the chances of the child falling into an extreme-risk group were high.

(Additionally, one cannot rule out possible genetic features in families or groups.) Studies on animals show that some strains are much more liable to opiate dependency than are others and that some strains are more responsive to amphetamines than are others. In humans, there is growing evidence for similar influences, for example, an inherited liver function such that alcohol is detoxified more slowly with the result that a greater and longer alcohol reaction takes place. Possibly other biochemical traits are inherited, linked to the preference for one or another drug or to the likelihood of particular kinds of reactions.

When one looks at population characteristics associated with use of drugs and with the risk of bad outcomes, it is often possible to identify important discriminating variables. Income levels are very important. This is seen in levels of use of psychoactive drugs—either for recreational purposes or by prescription—that tend to increase with family income. For example, people who drink alcoholic spirits (as opposed to cheaper wine) regularly tend to be richer than those who do not. It is also the case that increased individual consumption of alcohol is directly related to the risk of either acute inebriation or, over the long term, events such as cirrhosis, accidents, arrests, suicide, "skid row" status, and the like. Yet these latter are not in fact characteristic of high-income drinkers but rather of low-income drinkers. Thus among heavy drinkers one distinguishes at least two patterns; those with heavy use but lesser risk of troubles and those with more troubles even with less use. The latter are likely to come from minority, central city, impoverished, and fundamentalist backgrounds, and are likely to be males. Increased income therefore accentuates use probabilities but "protects" against visibly troublesome outcomes. In earlier decades it was thought that alcoholism was a problem that could arise only after years of steady drinking; that view has now been revised. Recent observations show that alcoholism embraces a variety of different problems and that many of these afflict not only people in their twenties, but teenagers and preteen children who also can and do have both acute and chronic drinking problems.

Other population data suggest that the percentage of problems with alcohol increases as the average per capita consumption of that drug increases. It is likely that this applies to other substances besides alcohol. If city A has an average of twice as much drinking as neighboring city B, then it is likely also to have more than twice as much alcohol troubles. Yet here, too, one must distinguish patterns, for in addition to level of consumption there are other trouble-determining factors. For example, regular alcohol use associated with dining, as when wine is consumed with a meal, is not only less likely to yield any problem (because, in part, wine tends to be metabolized differently than spirits and because the effects are modified when food is taken at the same time), but the style of use, as when taught to children, tends to insulate those children from later-life alcoholism. Examples of this are found among certain ethnic groups. For example, Greeks, Italians, and Jews use alcohol in social groups where authorities (parents) are present and learn what is expected in terms of self-controlled, proper behavior. Excess, rebellious, or other problem-expressing symbolic conduct in association with liquor is discouraged, as is the risk-taking drinking one finds among teenagers who learn their drinking in cars or back alleys. Thus one can have two cultures where alcohol consumption per capita is the same, but in the culture where this socially integrated and situationally controlled drinking occurs as part of family and cultural patterns, there should be fewer short- and long-term alcohol problems than in the culture with a different drinking style.

This matter of learning how to use drugs in safe ways and using them in safer rather than less safe settings applies to all the normally used psychoactive substances. Generally the greater the situational freedom, defined both in terms of the lack of external restraints and internal discipline, the more varied the behavior that can be expected. For instance, even when very high dosages of opiates are given under medical supervision over a long period of time so as to produce a real physical dependency, outcomes such as addiction, delinquency, or side effect illnesses are rare. When such controls are absent and, further, when the meaning of the experience changes, as occurs when youngsters use opiates as a means of pleasure seeking or as a means for proving their daring, then the chance for a problem increases even if the actual dosage of the drug is much less than in a medical situation.

The significance of such findings for the classroom is two-fold. Not only may it be worthwhile for students to learn the circumstances for the safer use of drugs—physician- or parent-supervised use is safer than peer use or solitary play—but the classroom itself becomes a possible instrument where safeguarding controls are learned, perhaps independently of the communication of knowledge about such things as socially integrated drinking. If, during the course of teaching, norms can be established which the children make part of their own beliefs and personalities (for example, norms which value self-control and limit use to approved situations), then the school itself and classmates there should become a standard of reference for what one ought and ought not do. This is one of the theoretically derived goals of what is called "process" drug education, where through discussion it is hoped that controlling norms will be established, ones that will be linked both to authority (the teacher and school and what they stand for) and to what peers learn to expect from one another. The experimental problem, of course, is to see if that process works. It is testable enough in terms of whether or not school authorities and peer norms are able to prevent prohibited forms of drug use from occurring in the school. It is another thing to test for effectiveness outside the classroom, where direct supervision does not occur.

The major epidemiological finding of the last decade is that the use of psychoactive substances is spreading. Spread is occurring in at least six directions. One direction is downward by age. That means that younger and younger people are using substances which were formerly the preserve of their elders. In the early 1960s marijuana and LSD were used by graduate students, in the mid-1960s by college juniors and seniors, and shortly thereafter by freshmen, followed more quickly by high school students; now, in metropolitan centers particularly, these drugs are used by grade school children. As our data will show, 10 percent of our samples report cannabis use and 7 percent report use of more exotic substances by the 6th grade. Already in the 2nd grade we have children reporting the use of alcohol and tobacco, whereas the first cannabis and inhalant use appears to have occurred in grade 4. California appears to be the pace setter for illicit drug use, but probably not for alcohol and tobacco. Quite likely there are other schools in other communities where the age levels for initial, unsupervised, nonprescription use of drugs is even earlier.

Another direction of spread is geographically outward. Outward means from metropolitan centers to small towns to rural areas, or within a city from the confines of one neighborhood spreading to other districts. Over the last fifteen years "outward" has usually meant outward either from experimental centers such as the San Francisco Bay Area with its early hallucinogen fashions, or from New York with its long-ensconced heroin neighborhoods, first to other metropolitan regions and thence to intermediate regions. In 1975, as federal authorities watched over heroin epidemiology, the expansion from cities to towns was becoming evident, just as the same process had been observed in England some eight years earlier.

A third spread is from one social class to another. When it was first used, LSD was restricted to upper middle class professional people who had access to the drug via legitimate laboratories or clinics. It spread upward to wealthier clients and students and downward to lower middle, working class, and lower class people. (The class designations of yesterday's sociology are not so neat these days because one must find some term for the nonworking ex-middle class hippies and junkies who, while qualifying by economic measures as poverty stricken, may have elected their new life styles by choice and carry with them some of the values of their wealthier parents.) Conversely, marijuana use in western agricultural regions and border states was once restricted to poor agricultural workers or their Spanish-speaking slum cousins, while heroin was considered the drug of the disaffected urban delinquent poor. These drugs have now spread upward to the working middle and upper classes. Coincidental in time and person has been the upward spread of the heroin addict life style, including begging, theft, prostitution, shoplifting, and the like. In each case there is the democratization of drugs and sometimes delinquency across socioeconomic classes.

Another spread outward has been by sex. When heroin and marijuana use were customs of the dislocated poor, they were primarily male customs. Just so was alcoholism primarily a male phenomenon, and cigarette smoking was once for men only. But now one finds female users and problem users, and in student populations as many females as males use these substances. Under special circumstances female users may outnumber males; for example, tranquilizers are more often prescribed for women, and it has been claimed, but not demonstrated, that in some areas more middle class women than men use barbiturates without medical supervision. In our own schools, described in the following chapters, there are as many girls as boys using marijuana, amphetamines, barbiturates, and hallucinogens, and more girls than boys using sanctioned substances (alcohol and tobacco) and inhalants.

A fifth kind of spread of use has been in the multiplication of substances used by individuals, a phenomena referred to as polydrug or multiple-drug use. There are a variety of substances available to children and adults via medical prescription, in the drug store as over-the-counter medications, in retail outlets selling alcohol and tobacco products, and illicitly. This availability, coupled with the individual, social, and cultural factors which predispose to a general interest in drug taking, leads to experimentation with and employment of a variety of chemicals over a lifetime. Phases of use are age related. In given locales experimentation or regular use are linked to age, as are peaks of use (and stages of decline when they occur, for example, as with illicit drugs during the 1920s).

(Drug use can occur in connection with other kinds of conduct which are correlated in time and in etiology, that is, by shared origins. Some kinds of drug use and delinquency are closely related and can be predicted by knowing about such things as neighborhood, race, family integrity, school performance, and personality. Insofar as there has been an expansion of delinquency-producing factors in our culture (or perhaps, better said, a reduction in those features which encourage civilized behavior), then more young people will elect to engage in illicit activities among which is the use of illicit drugs. Similarly, insofar as social and family features destructive of mental health are widespread, then youngsters suffering emotional ill health and character disorders (the latter, in turn, linked to delinquency as well) are likely to employ psychoactive drugs for self-medication, as vehicles for the expression of their psychopathology, as a consequence of poor judgment, and the like.

Multiplication of use is encouraged by the substitutability of one drug for another. Many compounds have somewhat similar effects; thus one can sedate or relax oneself with over-the-counter sleep aids, with barbiturates, with tranquilizers, with cannabis, or with alcohol. Conversely, one compound can have several effects, depending on, for example, expectations, dosage, biological rhythms, or the drug effect suggestions offered by others. One may seek substitute effects not ordinarily envisioned by drug classification schemes. Thus, if one seeks "stimulation," one may get it from barbiturates, alcohol, amphetamines, coffee, antidepressants, cannabis, or hallucinogens. Each may be experienced differently, but the person who wants a mood change may find that each is pleasing in its own way. Multiplication of use is also encouraged because people sometimes find a sequence of drugs gratifying, the one to counteract or to potentiate the other. An amphetamine user who is "up" may want to come down with a barbiturate or vice versa. A drinker who wants to sober up may try to do so with coffee. An LSD user on a bad trip may take a strong tranquilizer. And sometimes a combination of drugs is judged to be better than one drug by itself; barbiturates and amphetamines together give some people a glow; heroin laced with a little strychnine seems preferable to some; coffee with Irish whiskey yields a pleasing Irish coffee. And finally, once one is interested in drugs and convinced they are pleasing, there is a general readiness to try something new. Or if one already has enjoyed a substance and it becomes unavailable or too hazardous or troublesome to obtain, then why not try another in its place? Methadone replaces heroin; alcohol may replace methadone.

The sixth spread is one of increased per capita consumption. Over the last years this has been worldwide for alcohol. In the United States, this has occurred for prescribed tranquilizers, stimulants, and other mood elevators (although amphetamines and barbiturates are now being prescribed less often). Cigarette consumption, after a drop for a time under the impact of health danger warnings, is now rising again, as is the rate of uptake of cigarette use by youngsters. Inferences from survey, economic, and arrest data suggest that hallucinogen and cannabis use have risen dramatically over the last decade, and heroin use has also risen. It had been proposed early in the 1970s that heroin use was dropping after all, but by 1975, epidemiological estimates showed that this was not the case. Over-the-counter drug sales have not risen as dramatically as have these prescription, recreationally licit, and illicit uses. There is no reason to believe that the trend, especially for calming drugs and those that are part of or assist in sociability, will diminish in the near future.

The implications of these six kinds of spread for the schools are clear. Our society is experiencing, and can expect to experience further, a declining age level for initial exposure to and experimentation with psychoactive drugs by children both outside of medical or parental supervision and under those authoritative auspices. We can expect boys and girls to be equally exposed and interested. We can expect children of all social classes to be interested. We can expect willingness to use substances now associated with "being delinquent" (alcoholic spirits, heroin, barbiturates, tobacco, and cocaine) to increase as delinquency itself increases and also as laws are changed so that such drug use is not condemned. We can expect those who do use drugs to use a greater variety of them, and, while developing preferences that vary by age, person, and place, for children and adults to substitute one drug for another. We can expect schools now in regions where drug use is limited to lose their inexperienced status. As use increases nationally and worldwide on a per capita basis one can also expect some increase in problems, especially among those not insulated by wholesome families, "straight" peers, and individual sense, self-discipline, and good mental health. One says "some" because widening experience also teaches accommodation. The middle classes have learned to drink fairly safely. LSD users learn how to handle "bad trips" without going to a hospital. Heroin "chippers" control their use of heroin without ever becoming addicts.

There is by no means agreement on when a drug "problem" exists. Sometimes a child will agree with the teacher or school administrator that he or she has a problem, as for example, when there is infection, accident, psychosis, arrest, or withdrawal symptoms. Often a user will not agree, for many drug problems are in the mind of the observer rather than the user. Whatever the educator thinks, the youngster who is an addict may tell us he is having more fun than ever before. The delinquent user may tell us to go to hell while he robs a purse or wallet, insisting that he is right and society wrong, and that it is all somebody else's fault anyway. And besides, drugs make him feel better. The dropout can insist that school is ridiculous and society more so, that the world that matters is inside himself in the drug pictures in his mind. The impulsive pleasure seeker may reinvoke the arguments of the old hedonist philosophers, reminding us that life is short, that he or she is having a ball, and that we, with our worries and controls, are the crazy ones. Many children will be doing just what the others do, trying new experiences as part of learning about the world and their reactions to it, playing at what will one day be their adult drug habits.

The adult observer who disapproves vocally of children's sampling from our culture's chemical cafeteria may well be telling them what they loathe to hear, which means they may not listen to or like it. The older the student is and the more invested in drug-using ways, the less likely that teacher and student will enjoy a congenial discourse. Our data on student reactions show that by the 11th grade most students have had a wealth of drug experience, and they usually react negatively to drug education. By contrast, in the 2nd, 4th, and 6th grades, when authority still matters and children need not justify their contrary ways to themselves and their peers, reactions to drug education are positive.

Arguments with students about whether their drug use is or is not a problem, is or is not a bad thing, arc probably rare, because most of the time the teacher will not know about the child's drug use. In our own study, we found that among a total of 94 percent of the high school student body using any psychoactive drugs outside of medical supervision, only 1.5 percent had records and comments from teachers or administrators which showed them as "users." Teachers may have had their private suspicions, but our guess is that the drug use of most students passes unnoticed by school authorities. Some correlates, such as being a troublemaker, are more readily visible.

What people think constitutes drug "abuse" and what they want to see done about the drug "problem" varies, like drug behavior itself, with individual and social characteristics such as age, religion, political ideology, education, income, the nature of one's associates, and the like. Whether one studies legislators, college professors, narcotics police, or opinion poll findings, one learns that viewpoints about drugs are predictable because they are part of the larger fabric of beliefs about what is right and wrong, about self-discipline and pleasure, and about what human nature is like and what government must do in response. One should not be surprised then, that just as the etiology of drug risk bears a strong relationship to neighborhood, peer, and family habits and beliefs, so too do judgments about others' drug use which are also formed in these same social contexts. In consequence, as children and teachers bring in diverse points of view, the school and the classroom become settings not only for drug education but also theaters for combat about beliefs. Such conflicts ought to be least likely when the drug behavior falls in the evident categories of illness or venality. There is not much disagreement when people discuss drug overdose deaths or the sale of heroin by habitual adult felons, or when the treatment of depressed patients with antidepressant drugs or the religious use of wine in the Mass is considered. In between, whether one is talking about the social use of alcohol or cannabis or about self-medication with over-the-counter tranquilizers, there is less homogeneity of opinion. As a result, unless one consciously avoids the issues by never defining the possible varieties of drug "abuse," one facet of drug education will be the teacher's readiness to anticipate diversity of opinion and to deal with it as a social reality.

A factor of special importance in shaping both drug views and educational policy is the prior drug experience of the audience. One can estimate approval and disapproval of drug use by youngsters on the basis of what they have already done. Youngsters tend to approve of the drug use they have already engaged in and to disagree with adults who disapprove of it.

The work of Jessor and Jessor (1974) is particularly important here for it shows that a number of developmental patterns are closely linked to drug use, and that, for a given age, one can make significant predictions about, for example, sexuality, academic performance, lying, cheating, fighting, and marijuana use, simply by knowing the alcohol drinking status. At whatever age adolescents move into the regularly drinking group these other attributes merge, so that by being a member of a group defined by its drug use, a number of other social behaviors, including the need for peer approval and drug-related beliefs, are predictable. Youngsters in the nondrinker status tend not to approve of drinking, not to have drinking friends, and not to be deviant. They change once they move into the drinker status, approving their own and other drinking behavior and becoming generally less conventional. This reduced conventionality (defined as increasingly valuing independence, being more socially critical, having greater tolerance for transgression and approval of problem conduct, having lower esteem for achievement and religion, and becoming more peer oriented) implies, with increasing age, greater conflict in both beliefs and behavior between these older drug-using youngsters and their parents and teachers who remain conventional or who, even if themselves unconventional, try to persuade the children to be what they, the authorities, are not. No wonder, then, that drug education in the high school classroom is futile, insofar as it brings together the teacher as the advocate of conventionality and the juvenile experienced in and justifying his own drug behavior and associated unconventionality, and therefore attempts to prevent that which has already occurred.

This is not to say there is never a time when drug users change their attitudes or habits. That does occur as they mature, obtain valued membership in conventional groups, experience religious conversion, or respond to bad experiences, some of which may lead to—or may be—treatment or jail. Drug and other delinquencies typically become less frequent after the teens and early twenties. Some of the most extreme users die young. But drug dealers tire of the hassle, drinkers can become more moderate as they grow older, and one sees former smokers becoming independent. Whether or not formal education contributes to this by early inculcation of conventional values, one cannot say. That uncertainty parallels questions about the deterrent effect of criminal law.

One should not assume that children's unconventionality, of which illicit drugs are a part, inevitably represents "rebellion," "alienation," or a "generation gap." To the contrary, what some youngsters do very much reflects what their parents have trained them to do. Our own work on drug risk shows this, and the work of Kandel and Lesser (1972) emphasizes it for fields beyond drug use. The likelihood is that children's and parents' values are close, although this does not mean approval for specific conduct. If, for instance, the parents encourage independence and self-realization, the child can pursue these in a variety of ways which the parents had not anticipated, illicit drug use being one. Even so, the very choice of drugs as an activity is likely to be based on the parents as models, for parents also use drugs, even though theirs might be alcohol and tranquilizers rather than marijuana. Similarly, even when the drug use of youngsters is learned among and supported by their peers, this is not independent of parental influence, for children choose their friends on the basis of family training. If parents lack care, or if severe conflicts within problem families lead to rebellious choice of peers, then age-mate friends are chosen independently. For deviant drug users, rebelliousness is a major trait (Smith, 1973).

For the average child, friends will come from families of like religious, socioeconomic, and educational backgrounds. This constellation of influences, of which the youngster's own personality is certainly a part, will affect the response to the educational enterprise itself. Coleman (1966) and also Jencks *et al.* (1972) have emphasized that what children bring to school is at least as important as the school itself in determining levels of achievement by time of graduation. Kandel and Lesser (1972) show that educational plans are set in concert with both parents and peers, with the parental and especially the maternal influence being the greater. Love and Kaswan (1974), after finding that children's behavior in school (both grades and conduct problems) is intimately linked to their family environments, conclude that "whatever the school program, it is doubtful that school training can be successful without substantial cooperation between the school and the home." Not only is what children do in school predictable from their family experiences, but what they do with what they are taught depends upon its pertinence for their ordinary living. These investigators add that what is "taught" at home or in school is not necessarily what is said.

If we extrapolate from these reports to speculate on the response of the child to drug education, we would expect that a youngster's attitude toward drug education will have at least two components. One would reflect the general acceptance or rejection of the life style goals (including health, delinquency, adjustment) which are implicit in ordinary drug education. If the parents and peers believe in school as such, then there ought to be an acknowledgment by the child of the propriety and good intentions of drug education in the schools. The other component ought to be the relationship between the child's already acquired drug use experience and what he or she perceives as the approval or disapproval of the teacher, i.e., what is really communicated about drug conduct. The stage is set for a situation in which the child agrees—because his parents have agreed and their ideas are now his—that the school ought to teach drug education. At the same time, however, if what is taught is in conflict with what the child is already doing or believes he knows, the child would dispute, disparage, or ignore the educational content. It is a conflict between an acceptance in principle but a rejection of specifics. The more involved the child is in drugs, then the more the conflicts and the more unpalatable drug education may be because there are more points (i.e., more kinds of drugs and associated conduct) where the youngster is already doing what he is being taught not to do.

Our own data are consistent with these speculations. As children grow older they are increasingly antagonistic to drug education at the same time as they are becoming more intense and varied drug users. That antagonism is not diffuse but specific; among the 580 11th grade youngsters replying to questions about their receptivity to drug education, 53 percent of the replies were critical of the content but only 6 percent of the replies were critical of the drug education teachers. By contrast, in the 6th grade, of the 376 youngsters replying, 5 percent of the replies were critical of the content and 3 percent critical of the drug education teachers. These results are compatible with the notion that children accept their learned-at-home agreement, in principle, with drug education, and do accept the teacher as a person doing his or her job. It may be defensive rejection of what is taught on the part of drug-experienced high schoolers as compared with acceptance by elementary school pupils. As to data on parents, a survey conducted in one of our townships showed that the majority of parents considered drug education an important goal.

Taken together, these findings argue that there will be support for drug education from the child himself, his peers, and his parents, but that this support is attenuated as youngsters become either drug experienced or antagonistic toward school as such. Drug education should be conducted with those children who have not yet become too old to accept it. That is indeed the essence of preventive intervention.

Love and Kaswan (1974) found that the adequacy of children's behavior adjustment in school is correlated with grades and activity ratings, and that behavior problems tend to grow worse and compound themselves as the child grows older, with subsequent poor school performance being assured. One can imagine how, for this group of problem children, escape from their increasing problems (e.g., their family, their school, themselves) would be attractive. Drug involvement in the company of associates with like troubles and dropping out of school could be seen as solutions. Such "solutions" can represent both the problem—unusual drug use—that drug education is asked to prevent and, insofar as the student is already either not responsive in class or not in class at all, the circumstances which make an educational impact through normal classes most difficult to achieve. Johnson's (1973) study of 2200 high school boys from widely separate schools affirms Jessor and Jessors' (1974) findings of a correlation between an increased range of drug experience and poor grades and delinquency. The latter is associated with truancy Johnson found dropping out to be more common among illicit drug users than among other children. Intelligence was also found to be lower for any psychoactive drug users as compared with nonusers.[a] A psychiatric study (Abruzzi and Abruzzi, 1975) of 1000 heroin-using middle class upstate New York youths indicated that deep involvement in heroin was accompanied by disaffection for school and disinterest in learning.

Smith (1973), in a study of 15,000 students in grades 4-12, found that rebelliousness toward rules and authorities was the best single indicator of subsequent illegal drug use. Classroom apathy and poor grades were also correlates. In terms of personality traits those children who lacked conscientiousness, dependability, striving for recognition, high goals, persistency, planfulness, efficiency, manneriness, and agreeableness were more likely to become illicit users. And in a Tempe, Arizona (Jenkins, 1973) study of 9th graders, regular drug users valued excitement and sexuality much more than did nonusers and valued obedience much less. Wechsler and Thom (1972), studying drinking in junior and senior high school, observed that the heavy drinkers, who were also much more likely to be illicit drug users, were less academically oriented, made poorer grades, had more personal problems, and engaged in antisocial activities such as theft and vandalism. They were also more distant from their parents and more influenced by friends similar to themselves. Deviant drug use is connected with nondrug delinquencies. There is a general relationship between delin-

---

[a]In college, illicit drug users perform as well or better than and are as bright or brighter than nonusers. These high school results might well be different in schools where the majority of the student body engaged in widespread drug use.

quency, antischool attitudes, and poor school performance. Delinquents tend to have low educational aspirations, dislike their teachers, and are grade retarded in comparison with nondelinquents (Nettler, 1974).

In our own earlier work we found that children from age thirteen onward who were in the high drug risk group were more often self-indulgent, self-concerned, peer and pleasure oriented, heedless of the rights of others, and more lacking in self-discipline. We note finally a study by Robins and Guze (1972) which reported that alcohol problems in the ghetto for blacks, as for whites, occur when children are "brought up in families that are broken, irresponsible, illegal and contain adults with drinking problems. Alcohol problems are also predicted by early school problems, delinquency and drug use."

The foregoing findings are consistent. They show that the intensity and variety of drug use among youths is correlated with being troubled, in trouble, and not doing well in school. The implications of these youths' likely disinterest in and rebelliousness toward school present a forbidding challenge to educators who are asked to apply the very mechanism—education—that these youngsters have already rejected or found uncongenial, to alter or reverse an important component in a developmental pattern which begins well before school and is generated by powerful forces outside of school.

It is overly ambitious to expect the school to combat the drug-engendering aspects of culture, commerce, social and family life, and individual personality. Insofar as one times school intervention to take place after use has begun, additional difficulties are imposed beyond those noted above. Drug use provides many satisfactions. The more involved a drug user is, the greater the number of gratifications which can be claimed. Although a novice may only say of marijuana that it is an "interesting" experience, the aficionado may insist that it is simultaneously relaxing, aesthetic, thought provoking, erotic, a social facilitator, and fashionable. The conviction that a drug is multiply rewarding makes it all the more difficult to change a habit once it has begun. Should that habit be immersed in social living with constantly reappearing cues or stimuli to use, and should there be any actual distress when the drug is not available, then changing a habitual practice is even more difficult.

The foregoing are all reasons why it is likely to be more difficult for drug education to control use among students who are already regularly involved in drug use than with those who are not yet involved. This is an argument for preventive rather than "corrective" efforts in the classroom, and for timing the effort for younger rather than older children. That timing will depend on the ages at which youngsters have access to and begin to use various substances in different neighborhoods served by a school.

It is, of course, easy both to oversimplify and to give up. It is oversimplification to speak of only a few patterns when there are many. Neither intensity nor variety of psychoactive drug use inevitably creates bad outcomes; to the contrary, there are many youngsters who use a variety of drugs, including illicit ones, in ways that are these days quite normal. One dare not uncritically deduce from the presence of certain habits, such as, those of the normal California high schooler's smoking, drinking, and enjoying of cannabis, the same dire predictions that emerge from Robins' study of children from poor disrupted families. On the other hand, one cannot ignore the general relationships which obtain between heavy involvement in drugs and preexisting, current, and likely future troubles in living. As Robins and Guze (1972) write, "If an attack on early school problems can reduce the frequency of problem drinking, a host of other ghetto problems may well decline in consequence." One might add to that statement that the presence of early drug use of an intense and risky nature is itself a key to the need for intervention via case finding and referral.

In summary, the research tells us that many different forces operate to generate drug use among children. There are many kinds of use and outcomes. Among youngsters, those most at risk of deep involvement in drugs and real troubles in association with that use are the children most difficult for the schools to reach and to change. The implication is, at least, to intervene early before antischool attitudes and drug use become fixed, and before absenteeism removes part of the target audience from the classroom. The research also reminds us that the multiple audiences within a school or class, characterized by their drug use and its many personal and social correlates, are not likely to have the same response to a given educational program. As a result, one cannot expect uniform instruction to be equally appropriate for each student. For those students in trouble with drugs, or making trouble, the strategy of prevention is clearly too late; for these the task is one of treatment. Since there is no reason to expect that corrective force can operate in the ordinary classroom, the alternative strategy of case finding (that is, problem child identification) and referral to intensive and personally tailored caring personnel is appropriate.

Because we know that most youngsters will normally grow up to become drug-using adults, the preventive strategy itself can have only limited realistic objectives. It can set out to control drug use in the school itself. It can seek to retard the initiation of use, in the knowledge that such data as exist tell that the later the onset of self-administered use the more moderate the drug-using career. A preventive strategy can also be selective, targeting on substances which are disapproved by most adults and which are thereby ones least likely to be adopted for use by normally developing youngsters. That selectivity may not be rational pharmacologically but it will at least be conventional. Later, as folk drug classification schemes themselves benefit from advancing scientific knowledge, as, for example, people grow more wary of tobacco and barbiturates and less wary of marijuana, what is conventional for adults may itself change. Drug education must keep in step with scientific knowledge. A strategy of prevention must be modest and based on awareness of the countervailing strength of the other forces—cultural, social, and personal—which generate drug use. The public school, as we know it can never be a powerful independent drug use influence. It can reasonably target highly disapproved particular compounds as requiring permanent rejection (e.g., amphetamines, heroin, inhalents). The school can also encourage controlled rather than extreme use of given substances such as alcohol by communicating knowledge of the conditions under which moderate use is learned and unsafe outcomes are avoided. Implicit in the preventive strategy are the notions of timing, audience and drug specificity, as well as control via delay, via channeling (to safer as opposed to less-safe substances), and via moderation and discretion through social and self-discipline.

3 Speaking of Education: Approaches

This chapter considers approaches to drug education. It makes reference to an abundance of essays and efforts, sampling from pertinent observations.

Of all the writers on drug education, Woodcock has offered some of the most important observations. Here is what he has to say.

We tend to turn to education as an instrument of social policy aimed at specific kinds of deviant or delinquent behavior, or specific forms of ill health, only after experience (bitter sometimes for those on the receiving end) has convinced us that neither direct deterrence, in the shape of the law, nor curative measures, in the shape of medical care, can exercise effective control. Had we an effective cure or prophylaxis for dental decay, would we spend so much time teaching children to brush their teeth? In the case of drug usage, especially that by children and adolescents, we seem to have begun to accept the ineffectiveness of law or medicine and have duly begun to turn to education. Though this may be an indication of our growing ability to love the sinner, our need to hate the sin is not abated. As our espousal of an educational approach has deprived us of the average drug user as an object to be alienated by legal or medical means, so we have turned on the drug dealer, the "trafficker," as a recipient of our thwarted sense of outrage. Is it a coincidence that, in both the United States and the United Kingdom, a growing emphasis on drug education as a preventive weapon has been accompanied by an increase in the severity of the legal penalties for dealing? The United Kingdom Misuse of Drugs Act, 1971, for example, introduced simultaneously two new features into British drug legislation: preventive education, and "possession with intent to supply" as a new offense, distinct from simple possession of a controlled drug and carrying much harsher penalties.

To deny, however, that education may have a role in the prevention of drug-using is to ignore our belief in the role of education as a road to the achievement of socially accepted lives and values and, particularly in the United States, as a means of homogenizing the population. To want to use education as a means of establishing desirable behavior and values vis-à-vis drugs is thus an expression of our confidence in the schools as molders of citizenship and inculcators of a kind of conformity.

Deciding on Drug Education

Preceding the adoption of education, there has been a debate, not about its efficacy, but about the direction of its impact. The question usually asked is not whether drug education in the schools has any effect, but whether it will lead to more rather than less drug use and, correlatively, greater or fewer drug-related problems, dealing included. It is thus apparent that the potency of the school as a force for affecting drug conduct is assumed. Although the debate has been resolved in the United States by assuming a favorable impact, the World Health Organization Expert Committee on Drug Dependence (1970) has concluded to the contrary and recommended against drug education. Inspection of the decision process indicates that drug education will be suggested only when the known prevalence of illicit or otherwise disapproved drug use among school-age youngsters has reached a level at which one need no longer worry that education will itself promote interest in use. This argument was made explicit by the chairman of the United Kingdom Health Education Council who stated in Parliament during a debate on the 1971 Misuse of Drugs Bill that the development of policy guidelines for schools on drug-abuse education must await the results of social surveys on youthful drug use (Birk, 1971).

Even in the absence of studies showing high prevalence, that is, illicit experience among the majority, for those nations where there is any indication that illicit use is occurring, there are pressures for the schools to take some action. Since direct education is forbidden until high prevalence levels are reached, the interim measure adopted most often appears to be an indirect one: the education of teachers so that they will at least be knowledgeable about drug problems and will be able, presumably, to intervene informally in special cases, as, for example, when children themselves raise questions about drugs or when a child is found to be a drug user.

There are conditions under which, even in the absence of high prevalence of use among school-age children, it is proposed that a second form of interim measure is required. These circumstances occur when it becomes apparent, either from scientific studies or official records, that adult use of illicit drugs occurs, that adult use is expanding, and that there is fear that children upon leaving school will be exposed to previously nonexistent drug-taking temptations. In such situations, proponents of education propose that the schools must intervene to forestall that possible future use. The formula most often advanced is that factual information about the effects and dangers of drugs will suffice to retard later experimentation.

The foregoing suggests three areas of decision. One is the level of risk of future use by adults, the second is a band frequency of unknown width when some children's use is occurring but is not yet deemed great enough to justify direct education, and the third is when a critical point of prevalence among children has been reached such that the risk of arousing interest is more than offset by the risk of not intruding to stabilize, if not to reduce, current use. Yet the prevalence is often a subjective estimate in the mind of the decision maker rather than the product of reliable data on levels and patterns of use determined scientifically. Thus if one introduces the notion of a critical mass of use required to produce pressures for drug education in schools, the mass may not be that which is found in the population itself but that which exists in the perceptions of those who influence school activities. The sources of such beliefs are varied; but, at the very least, they include highly publicized cases in the mass media, police alarms, parental anxiety over changing conduct styles among children, and school concerns over their institutional reputations for moral soundness. All these events occur on an international stage where the backdrop consists of the very active demons of popular drug mythology. Faced with perceived threats and such demons, the average citizen feels compelled to take some action. One of the most convenient pressure points is the school. As one English citizen wrote, after hearing a debate on the pros and cons of drug education, 'I am sure we must educate our young people about the dangers of drugs. At least we will have done our duty.'

Bureaucratization

Once a decision has been reached to introduce education, be that indirectly of teachers or to deter future use or more directly to affect present student habits, drug education itself becomes institutionalized and subject to the usual snowballing of bureaucratization. This means that there will be pressure for the evercreasing appropriation of funds, the emergence of a cadre of experts, the definition of sets of proper and improper techniques, including demands for personnel training and certification, competition with other subjects for the time of the school-child audience, competition among educational suppliers for the new market in teaching aids, and the growth of vested interests dependent upon the continued expansion of this particular industry. Bureaucratization very early reaches the point at which, given the current politics and demonology of drugs, it is irreversible.

Philosophy

What is done by way of drug education will reflect how teaching is conducted generally in a society. This in turn rests upon views as to the nature of man and the particular nature of children. In those fields of instruction bearing on social conduct and self-control, as does education in the drug field, it is pertinent to ask if the society regards the child as inherently sinful or angelic, as a tabula rasa, or as a prize or chattel.

In the Western world, certainly England of yesteryear, the view was that children were born bearing the sins of the father and thus had devilish potential (not unlike current Balkan peasant beliefs to the effect that the unbaptized child is a drak, or demon). Education therefore had to instruct for enlightenment and to control the powers of darkness. It was consequently moral in tone, civilizing with respect to aims, and repressive or controlling in classroom practice. Drug education in such cases should be in the context of ethics, an exhortation to elect nonuse as good and godly, the warning that use is evil, and the practice of strong punishment should the discovery of drug use be made.

Belief in the child's nature as essentially neutral, that is, a tabula rasa, pretends to be an areligious doctrine. From it one would expect the educator to assume the child pliable and in need of molding, probably through facts and by good example. Bad influences such as the "wrong" information or bad companions are to be avoided lest proper development be impaired. The term proper is probably defined by community norms, religious though these may be; but the educator, preferring to be "objective," elects to see himself as a pragmatist working to avoid harm. That concept of harm can be described in physical, social, or mental terms and, like the mental health movement, it conveys much that is conventional under a scientific disguise.

The angelic child, lineal descendent of the noble savage of Rousseau, seems to be growing in popularity, especially in America, although Summerhill in England is a prototype. The modern belief may represent in part some misreading of Freud, an adaptation of the psychodynamic commentary on repression as a dangerous force leading to neurosis, the result of which must then be avoidance of repression, currently expressed as aversion to control. For Freud, of course, the savage was not so noble, discontent being, for him, a necessary outcome of the forces required to build a working conscience. Nevertheless, the current interpretation would see oppressive society as the source of discord juxtaposed against the child's innate harmony with nature. Parents do wrong to destroy this natural harmony through coercion; so also do educators who thus sense that they must instead beckon rather than compel. The drug educator proceeding according to this assumption must be sure not to restrain or antagonize; such actions as he takes must aim only to arouse and channel the natural interest of the child or, in the extreme form, pander to his desires.

Approaches

The Health Approach. There are several alternatives by which drug education may find its niche in school systems. By far, the commonest is to consider drug education a form of health education. The assumptions here are that drug use is a health problem, that is, its occurrence represents some form of illness—mental or physical—and that this illness is preventable by supplying appropriate information. A similar model is venereal disease education. Accident and dental caries prevention programs are also similar. Such health models may be employed even if it is recognized that some forms of drug use are not in themselves evidence of illness; casual cannabis smoking can be an example. However, such drug use is always held to present the risk of a future health problem so that the health model approach is sustained.

Both assumptions underlying the health approach are of course in doubt. The contention that ill health is demonstrable simply by fact of drug use is strongly questionable. Whether or not preventive programs work in any area of health education is also dubious. Controlled studies of such programs are rare and their results tend to be discouraging, even when the chosen objectives and target populations would seem almost to guarantee success. For example, Schlesinger and others (1966) used intensive programs involving discussion groups, specially appointed block leaders, visiting experts, and monthly newsletters—all aimed at teaching parents of children under seven how to protect them from accidental injury with no discernible effect whatever. Similarly, Adams and Stanmeyer (1960) found that, in a group of United States servicemen in Antarctica, films and lectures had no significant impact on dental self-care; only close individual supervision by a dentist made any difference. Neither of these studies was aimed directly at children, but dare we build upon the hope that children will respond more rationally to health education than do their elders?

The Delinquency Approach. Illicit drug use among children is necessarily a matter of delinquent conduct; it is a failure of children to be law-abiding. Search reveals remarkably few programs designed to inculcate law-abiding conduct as such, leaving aside recourse to punishment or corrections after the fact. One such teaching program in California employed in grades 7 and 8 seeks to instill understanding of the basis and nature of the criminal law. In the United Kingdom, Hauser (1963) has sought to encourage a sense of relationship to society and the law among adult offenders, and recently to inaugurate similar programs preventively in the school.

Were such programs to be employed more widely, the outcomes might be in doubt. An intensive effort to prevent vocation, school, and law-abiding failure has been reported by Ahlstrom and Havighurst (1971). The study began with socially disadvantaged youngsters in the seventh grade for whom the prognosis for vocational, school, and lawful adjustment was lower than ordinary (given statistics on their predecessors and peers). The investigators worked with the group through high school, studying their total environment and trying out a work-study program. A control group received regular academic work whereas the experimental group received considerable extra vocational and counseling services. The extra effort made no difference, measured statistically, although one-fourth of the boys were presumed to have profited in one fashion or another. The majority of the experimental sample ended up socially and educationally maladjusted and with a record of continuing delinquency. Drug use as such was not recorded, but it is reasonable to expect that this group that was so widely involved in crime—including homicides and rapes—would not have overlooked pharmaceutically derived peccadilloes.

Social Learning. In communities in which drug use by children has become so widespread as to be statistically normal and, to some extent, accepted as inevitable by authorities, one can distinguish another approach, one that is less well elucidated because it does not subscribe to the traditional health or delinquency definitions of drug use, although it may incorporate these. In California, for example, where in metropolitan areas the majority of youngsters over age 12 admit to at least experimentation with cannabis, several school systems experiment with programs based on the assumption (empirically supported) that most drug use by children cannot be demonstrated to have immediate or long-term health hazards (for example, cannabis experimentation) nor need it be associated with nondrug delinquency (R.H. Blum, 1972, personal communication). Since the origins of this behavior are complex, arising from child-rearing styles (Blum and Associates, 1972b), and are dependent upon opportunities for access to drugs among peers, the goals for school intervention are limited. It is assumed that education cannot affect the on-going illicit drug behavior (including alcohol and cigarette use) that is normally learned (from peers, from advertising, in consequence of parental values and conduct, and the like) but that it may conceivably either prevent or reduce the unusual drug use that has demonstrably greater risks for health, arrest, social adjustment, and so forth (for example, self-injection, glue-sniffing, unsupervised drinking of hard liquor, and barbiturate use). One goal is to create among children new group norms that operate to control these abnormal uses; another is to deflect whatever emotional or symbolic processes may lead certain children to unusual, dangerous-drug use.

Techniques. What goes on within the classroom depends not only upon the model employed for describing drug use and upon the goals set (prevention, encapsulation, reduction; general for all drugs, specific for drugs or manner of use) but also upon the teaching methods believed to be most efficacious—or perhaps simply most convenient. Techniques vary as to the intensity of application—whether one hour per year or one hour per week—and the teaching materials and styles employed. It appears that at present there is great reliance on teaching aids—manuals, film, and other teacher-supplementing devices. Perhaps some of the popularity of teaching aids may be attributable to the uncertainty of teachers themselves as to how or what to teach, given their own lack of training in this field, the alternative models, and the frequent absence of clearly explicated goals.

Whether or not the uncertainty one postulates for teachers in this difficult role also arises from doubt about the efficacy of traditional didactic approaches is unknown. Certainly the teacher called upon to give just the facts may be expected to have some doubts about it, if only because the two groups of people most knowledgeable about drugs also seem to have very high risks not just of use but of demonstrable poor outcomes. These are, among the "respectable," physicians, and, among young people, the drug dealers themselves.

As soon as teachers consider moving away from a traditional didactic approach, they are also likely to be assailed by doubts, this time about their competence in this more ambiguous situation to handle matters of values, symbols, emotions, and social rather than school learning. Most are equipped neither by training nor by disposition to set foot in this poorly charted terrain (Aubrey, 1971).

One development, which seeks both to replace didactic method with one allowing more feedback from the consumer himself—the school child—and at the same time to provide a modicum of structure for the teacher, is variously called group counseling or process education. It is one of the components of the drug education experimental design in San Mateo county. At its very simplest, it substitutes give-and-take discussion for information-giving by the teacher. At a more complex level, it can be seen as a method using group dynamics to instill new group norms regarding drug use; while, as counseling, it may be expected at least to divert individuals with demonstrable maladjustment away from symbolic and emotional investments in dangerous forms of drug use as "solutions" to their difficulties. But again, if all the evidence for psychotherapy over these many years is so equivocal as to success, dare the schools hope for better through process education?

The Moral Approach. Whether explicitly considered a matter of health, crime, social learning, or what-have-you, it has long been evident that moral judgments play a strong role in describing drug use. The word abuse makes that clear enough. Similarly, such studies of the etiology of illicit use as exist make it clear that values and beliefs do have strong predisposing functions. It can be assumed that regardless of the label under which the schools present their endeavor, all parties to it recognize that drug education is partly a moral endeavor. The explicitness with which this is acknowledged varies with cultural context and, one suspects, specifically with the religious orientation of school and community. Had there been drug education a hundred years ago, it is likely that the moral approach would have been primary, as indeed it usually was in education about alcohol at the time. Today, in countries in which traditional religious morality is taught in the schools, we may expect that drug education will be subsumed under religious ethics. Under these circumstances, disapproved drug use is bad—and, in Christian lands, sinful. The educational prescription is to say No. For the young children, that formula is not only appropriate in terms of Piaget's observations on the moral development of children but, given an integrated and supporting community, probably effective as well. On the other hand, under conditions of social change or of family or individual psychopathology, one would expect that the cost of repressive moral education can include some extreme counterresponses. If, for example, as with sex, there is a powerful natural urge toward altered states of consciousness—attainable perhaps most readily through drugs—then one would expect unhappy long-term consequences from the simple repression of drug use unless other rituals existed for producing altered states or unless sanctioned situations for ritualized drug use were present.

Accepting Altered States. The thesis that altered states of consciousness are widely sought and enjoyed and constitute natural biological as well as perhaps spiritual phenomena is advanced by Weil (1972). In support of Weil, one may observe the propensity of cats to get stoned on catnip, of children to engage in the Valsalva maneuver, and of almost all cultures so far described to use one or another psychoactive drug for nonmedical purposes. Weil, along with Meher

Baba, William James, Saint John of the Cross, and Lord Buddha, would maintain the necessity as well as the value of the experience of altered states of consciousness. Weil proposes that, insofar as drug use is an attempt to satisfy this human potential, either drug use or alternatives for reaching altered states should not only be condoned but should be actively taught to children. Should his proposals be put into effect, drug education would consist of teaching meditation and, insofar as drugs were involved, the safe use of drugs as ancillaries. Such drug education or its prototypes may already occur in certain spiritual communities or in those hippie families where children are early initiated into drug use. Since the Manson "family" may also be taken as an illustrative case, we trust that the proponents of Weil's scheme would attend to suitable support and control structures.

Community Centers. Schools can be the center of drug education efforts while shifting their emphasis from the teaching of children—or teachers—to that of becoming a community resource. In such a situation, the school becomes a center for activities as well as learning, a place where parents come for drug information or counseling, where cases of unusual or dangerous forms of drug use by children are identified and referred to professional or other helping sources, and where outreach programs begin. In the community survey conducted by Blum and his associates (1972a) as part of their family studies, parents and drug-responsible professionals not only nominated education as the most desirable form of intervention with regard to drug problems, but seemed most willing to use the school as the central community resource.

Focus

For the most part, existing and planned drug education programs have focused on the illicit or exotic drugs, have been aimed at all rather than some students, have opted to present information but not to handle cases, and have remained safely obscure in offering general goals (drug-abuse prevention) rather than specific ones. Each of these quite understandable developments may be taken as a problem in its own right or, put differently, as an opportunity for future development.

The emphasis on illicit and exotic drugs is to the exclusion, in many places, of those most widely employed substances, alcohol and tobacco, with their quite noticeable burden of immediate and long-term adverse effects. Yet, whether one is concerned with the prevention of these effects (alcoholism, assault, road accidents, upper respiratory infections, heart disease, and lung cancer) or on the very specific prevention of that drug problem par excellence, drug dealing, it would appear that the focus must include alcohol and tobacco. Consider the finding in *The Dream Sellers* (Blum and Associates, 1972b) to the effect that the earliest and most wide-spread admission of anxiety over a drug problem on the part of the young dealers was in connection with their drinking. Even if these already or soon-to-be drug-peddling youngsters were using cannabis, LSD, amphetamines, or opioids, it was their alcohol use that they could first see—or admit to seeing—as presenting a problem to them. This being so, it would follow that drug education in schools might well consider safe and unsafe forms of drinking and, in essence, teach the safer uses (at home, under supervision, with meals, wine or beer rather than spirits, and so forth) before as well as during adolescence.

The danger signals for alcohol problems might also be taught, not just for self-recognition but for helpful use with friends and family as well. Indeed, this option gives to alcohol and tobacco a most favored place in education, since inquiry about and discussion of them in class need evoke no fear of the police or of the narcotics laws operative in all nations that subscribe to the Single Convention. Some students, beginning most often in the mid-teens if the data of Blum and his associates (1972a) are generalizable, will recognize themselves as already in the danger-signal category. Clearly, the giving of information will only affirm what they fear, and that affirmation must be done in a way that allows constructive action to be taken. The question, for these youngsters who identify themselves as cases, is: What is to be done?

At this point, the general focus of the schools might well be replaced with a more individualized one, and the information-giving function might be supplemented by systematic case finding and referral. Such steps imply considerable expansion of the facilities for helping children and adolescents. The needs for personnel and facilities in the United States are well documented by the recent report of the Joint Commission on Mental Health of Children (1969) and their inadequacy in the United Kingdom has been described by Payne (1971). Lest the drug-using youngster be given attention to the exclusion of the child who suffers other problems of living and lest the latter be forced into taking or pretending to take drugs in order to qualify for treatment, it is imperative that such child-care facilities be general rather than drug-specific.

The foregoing focuses imply specification of goals in drug education by drug, by individuals, by developmental status, and by community as opposed to the amiable but simplistic drug-abuse prevention now advocated. Such tailoring is predicated on the existence of and knowledge about diversity of forms of drug use among children and youth as well as follow-up data that enable one to say which forms of drug use are likely to be benign and which dangerous. It also assumes the availability of different approaches to individuals or groups of users depending upon their stage of life and their drug habits. It further assumes some knowledge about the relative efficacy of one or another form of intervention to be applied in school to these different consumers of school drug programs.

Evaluation

The extent of drug education has tended to be inversely related to the degree of evaluation. This is perhaps not accidental, given the degree of disquiet that evaluation efforts can arouse in the hearts of those with vested interests. Indeed, any demonstration of the inefficacy of drug education could hardly be welcome by anyone who has dedicated hopes or career to drug education for itself. Yet a note of optimism may be injected. In the United States, there is massive drug education with now, belatedly, the small beginnings of evaluation. In the United Kingdom and Holland, there is some drug education with proportionately much more (though still not much) accompanying outcome evaluation. In Australia, drug education evaluation precedes, in pilot-project form, any commitment to drug education per se. This progression, temporal and geographical, in the emphasis placed on evaluation is welcome evidence that the voices crying in the wilderness for education based on demonstrable results are finally heard. Nevertheless, insofar as evaluations that are under way are examining only attitudes and intentions, not drug use and outcomes, such efforts are insufficient. Perhaps direct measures are allowable only in those communities in which drug use has already achieved a high level of prevalence. That being so, this constitutes an argument for the correlation of attitude and intention measures with actual manner of drug use and their outcomes. It also is an argument for concentration in education and evaluation on the prevention (and individualized case referral) of dangerous alcohol and cigarette use. Such programs should also be accompanied by research in a variety of environments on the relationships between such approved drug use (in Western countries) and disapproved use including the particular related problem of drug-dealing.

Let us assume that reliable large-scale research were to tell us that drug education in the schools is essentially worthless as far as affecting the drug use and drug-use outcomes of children. What then? The most likely answer is that drug education would continue, the evaluators would be fired, and whatever methods they used to achieve such calamitous findings would be ridiculed. Such an eventuality may be taken as just retribution on the evaluators for having taken a narrow view, construing the purpose of their evaluation to be to pronounce moral judgment of a yes/no variety on the goodness of education rather than to use evaluation as an opportunity to learn more about the impact of teaching and to feed back this knowledge into schools, teaching them how better to proceed. The firing of evaluators may also be taken as just retribution for their having assumed the major motive of drug education simply to be to change drug behavior of children, rather than comprehending it as an expression of the intense need of people to act "for the good" despite uncertainty of how that good may be achieved. One has in mind the insightful work of E. and J. Cummings (1957) showing how the best-intentioned community mental health program defeated its own ends when it failed to understand the dynamics of existing institutions, processes, and beliefs in a community.

The more evaluation can be seen as an integral component of drug education rather than a one-shot alien process, the more likely it will be to yield insights applicable to achieving the several ends implicit and explicit in drug education. Educational evaluation must be akin to engineering developmental design with its continuous process of feedback and modification. It must not use as a model the laboratory test of the null hypothesis whereby the observing scientist, uninvolved, negates the life work of his fellows.

It will be seen that two further opportunities lie herein. One is that insights developed through evaluation may be used to assist citizens over time to think through their goals for their children and for their schools and thus refine them, perhaps making constructive use of that contradiction inherent in much of the current scene. The other opportunity is for research personnel to treat this scheme as a clear invitation to join the ever-growing pyramid of bureaucrats who justify themselves on the basis of their existence and not their accomplishments. This dilemma has yet to be resolved.[a]

A number of writers, and following them a number of programs, have considered what the content of drug education might be. Like Birdwood (1972), most acknowledge, implicitly at least, the likelihood that the wrong approach to drug education may, as Woodcock also implies—be harmful. Hammond (1972), for instance, has called attention to the "catastrophe" represented by the fact that most educational materials evaluated by the National Education Association have been judged to be "false, poor, emotionally oriented and (narrowly) judgmental, more harmful than no material at all."

[a]Reprinted with permission from *Drug Dealers, Taking Action*, Richard Blum and Associates, San Francisco: Jossey Bass Publishers, (1973).

Process Education

To avoid such content failures and to emphasize the full range of events occurring in the child which lead to drug abuse, a number of commentators have proposed alternatives which go well beyond the giving of facts (or, often, misinformation). Bedworth and D'Elia (1971) have emphasized helping the individual decision making process. Weinstein and Brayer (in Faber, 1973) have offered a carefully constructed program, evaluated by Carney (1970 a,b) with special attention to risk taking propensities, based on the concept of value clarification. Kurzman (1974) has reported on a communication skills seminar as an alternative, whereas Dohner (1972) has proposed that alternatives to drug use through exercises in personal awareness can be taught. Faber (1973), citing Newington, concentrates on a mental health approach which seeks to build self-esteem. Clark's (1972) "Operation Future" stresses positive value development in children. Slimmon (1973), in an "alternatives and values clarification" effort, strives to create conscious awareness of alternatives to drugs for pleasure and mood change, to increase value system clarity and rational decision making, to enhance self-esteem, to provide adult models who can be respected, and to form peer groups with non-drug-taking norms. The Michigan Department of Education program (1973) has much the same broad themes, including help in self-direction and problem exploration and children's participation in drug information evaluation itself. The Michigan guidelines also stress the importance of the teacher's orientation and personality, for it requires teachers who are well adjusted, flexible, credible, and who enjoy excellent rapport with students. Yolles (1971) has also underlined the need to select and train teachers carefully for such programs. Poliakoff (1971) has suggested a program for that training. Feinglass' (1969) NIMH-supported training center is an example of a very comprehensive training effort. Einstein *et al.* (1971) also describes a careful teacher training program which stresses the selecting of teachers in advance if they are to benefit and if the programs are to be well conducted.

Segal (1972) does not deemphasize information giving, but describes how discussions of information itself can incorporate the importance of attitudes and, more broadly, the relationship of people's use of drugs to social issues. In doing so, medical, psychological, legal, moral, and religious aspects would necessarily be considered. Schwartz (1974) in a short but powerful paper goes further, contending that school programs aimed at high-risk youngsters—he estimates 15 percent are in that group—would begin, anticipating developments for several decades later, with family planning courses and demonstration teaching of child development and care. There would be obligatory parental guidance and education for children in trouble and those cases would be identified beginning in kindergarten. There would be integrated use of community resources and, in school and out, counseling for the child and parents. Vocational training at a later date would help make education meaningful but would be designed to assist self-esteem. The educational system itself would become more humanistic, making a central theme of training children to themselves become parents and making the schools available to contemporary parents to assist them in their child rearing.

The twentieth technical report of the World Health Organization's Expert Committee on Drug Dependence (1974) proposes expanded responsibilities for schools, differentiating between teaching (information giving) and education. The latter is a broad effort to shape children by all influences available within the school, selecting both audiences and methods on the basis of the administrators' and teachers' knowledge of the etiology of various drug problem patterns and the likely development of various life styles among children with particular backgrounds and dispositions. The WHO report incorporates or implies much that is contained in existing programs that go beyond fact giving. As with Hess (1972), these commentators are aware that the rational model which sees a developing child as capable of making "decisions" about drugs is insufficient; this is more true the younger the child, and the more so when he or she is already subject to strong forces which reduce the freedom of choice (if one uses a free will model at all), so that what happens in the drug sphere is determined by events quite beyond the child's control.

De Lone (1972), in a concise analysis, considers some of these same problems juxtaposed to the perspective the high-risk child has of the school, and he writes: "Schools . . . frequently promote the kind of life style that is anathema to drug abusers; conformity, authoritarianism, a certain rigidity"; he adds what we noted earlier, that they are, to boot, at best a modest influence compared with home, peers, and neighborhood. De Lone proposes that if one examines the drug education problem one finds that it is the school's problem: "drug abuse is a peculiar microscope magnifying many of the flaws in education . . . that reformers have carped about from Rousseau to Silberman. It is precisely for this reason that the drug issue has potential to become a powerful lever for school reform." In consequence, the main tasks "would be to create a new school culture, one that provides a significant alternative to the drug culture . . . this means no less than fundamental institutional change." De Lone holds that schools cannot prevent drug abuse by teaching about it but "they are not helpless to alleviate it." He suggests there be emergency procedures including crisis intervention, that no school have as a goal drug use prevention, and that schools ignore recreational users and concentrate on finding and dealing with high-risk children. Among the methods employed in New York City to do this are directed rap sessions with ensured confidentiality that provide a sanctuary for working out troubles, the use of temporary alternative schools with a specially selected counseling roles, and the involvement of students in designing and evaluating their own drug programs.

Tresan, in his (1972) report on a San Francisco school project run by psychiatrists, distinguishes two models which can be applied after one has decided to go beyond the facts. The medical model calls for the identification and treatment of particularly distressed persons through special handling and referral, much as in the De Lone New York program. This mental health model, not unlike the proposals of Schwartz earlier noted, provides for extra services outside of class to a select student population. This approach need not use drug problems as its criteria for case finding, although given the high correlations between drug problems and other difficulties in adjustment, school performance, and delinquency, one would certainly expect that problem drug use is as good as any known criterion by which to identify children in need of extra help. Once an administrative decision has been made and implemented to employ the mental health referral model, then programs of the sort described by Cowen (1971) can be inaugurated.

The other model which Tresan describes is essentially that of humanistic psychology and embraces much that commentators such as Weil (1972), Dohner (1972), and Slimmon (1973) propose. As Tresan states, "the ultimate problem is not one of suppressing a given behavior so much as promoting an enhanced sense of life and relatedness to others." To do this the school must offer "due consideration for the overall well-being of its students." In terms of classroom planning Tresan requires three prerequisites:

The first is that it be based on highly individualized relationships and relevant occurrences rather than on a set format designed to inculcate a body of generalized impersonal facts. Secondly, and this flows from the first consideration, the participants and instructor of such a class in order to attain some trust of one another must be together over a relatively long duration of time. (A minimum of 25 hours meeting time would seem necessary. This is a rough estimate based on my knowledge of group phenomena.) Thirdly, the instructor must understand how to facilitate group interactions, but more than this, he must resemble in attitude the "rogue-teacher" of which George Leonard writes in his book *Education and Ecstasy*. This is a person who through his own well-considered experiences has come to regard all human behavior, delinquent though it may first appear, as potentially instructive and edifying. In short, he need allow experiences in life to happen without condemning them, but help at the same time to give some coherence and meaning to those experiences. He must be ready to see the searching and floundering in the drug-abusing youth, not just the reprehensible and dangerous aspects. He must allow students to struggle with moral issues, and yet be bold and comfortable enough to inquire and examine. He must be aware of the age-specific developmental tasks that the students face, such as increasing independence from family, peer acceptance and conformity, learning about intimacy and sex, and career considerations. He must be willing to help explore personal reactions to these developmental problems, such as moodiness, anger, boredom, thoughts about death or meaninglessness of life, and of course, aberrant behavior.

The approach of Tresan, combining humanistic hopes with psychodynamic understanding, is rather more open ended in method and aims than traditional didactic teaching or the guided format of decision making or other process education forms. Both of these latter approaches, unlike Tresan's developmental facilitation, rest heavily on the assumption that children are rational creatures who, given particular information, will decide on their own not to use drugs in a way which disturbs their elders.

A contrary assumption is made by Zinberg et al. (1976), whose approach to drug education is psychoanalytic. They argue against any information programs whereby the teacher seeks to impose a goal on children, as, for example, avoidance of drug abuse. They contend that by insisting on rationality one does not dissipate ever-present irrationality and that the most effective approach to this human complexity is not direct, didactic, or immediately practical. These clinicians observe that information reception is not a passive activity; instead there is selective perception and repression "into myths or misconceptions" in keeping with emotional relations. There has usually been no lack of information in children's lives and so the question is: Why do they act as they do? It is because information about salient matters—in this instance morality, pleasure, adulthood, etc., all linked to drug conceptions—is subject to unconscious psychodynamic forces which distort information processing. What education must do, they argue, is allow children to explore why it is they do not use more information more clearly, a discussion process which appears to require a well-integrated, mature, nonmoralizing, psychodynamically sensitive teacher. Any other effort in "an attempt to shape the opinions and judgments of its students . . . is potentially an instrument of regimentation and reduces rather than increases the individual's capacity to choose." Since, they claim, there are but drug facts to be communicated, ordinary drug education is in fact "social indoctrination," communicating the "righteous moral imperative, of 'No.' "

Zinberg et al.'s alternative provides two kinds of training: one to "help teachers identify and work through the interpersonal factors affecting their ability to teach and cope with their classes"; and for children, discussions to "teach young people that they can communicate with each other about topics and feelings usually kept to oneself . . . " with the aim of making "members sufficiently aware of their own unconscious motivations and sensitive to the feelings of others to permit more rational reality testing." In addition, consultation to school superintendents is provided. The method of group leadership does not encourage conformity but seeks to generate ego-autonomous action, that is, enlightened, integrated self-control, a maturity which stands against both inner impulsivity and external temptation or force. Such other-respecting independence would mean, Zinberg et al. acknowledge, that children would become more exploratory. In the drug arena the inference is that they would expand their use of nonharmful psychoactive drugs, regardless of conventional strictures.

Advocates of both didactic and process teaching, including value clarification, are more optimistic than Zinberg et al. about the cognitive capacities of children in relation to self-control and the worth of directed education.

Both methods posit that there is, or can be created, a conscious set of steps through which children, once drugs become available to them, can begin to weigh facts about these substances, can make risk and benefit estimates as to effects on their own lives, and can then proceed to act, regardless of other influences, on this conscious decision. The usual educational goals also imply, but do not state, that the facts given will be weighed heavily on the negative side; that is, that the scientific evidence will be compellingly antidrug when considered by a reasonable child. Such assumptions about rationality, about conscious decision making, and about the nature of objective drug information are at best dubious. As we shall see, the evidence as to the effects of such programs does not encourage these assumptions.

It is not unlikely that educators who advocate such programs would also grant that other processes may also be at work in the classroom. In process education there may be group dynamics at work such that new peer group norms are set up which become informal group controls over drug use. One would also expect that a teacher who is an admired and credible person would become a model to be followed. And, in teaching, when fear is aroused it can have a deterrent effect, at least for the short term. Yet these possible influences seem to be considered as subsidiary, in the service of drug education per se. The most common assumption is that drug conduct is best shaped in the schools by trying specifically to influence children's thinking about drugs. A partial exception occurs in value clarification approaches where one seeks to focus on the decision process itself, on value development or identification, and on risk taking propensities as such. Drugs are then introduced as the arena where choices can be identified. The teaching goal in value clarification remains that of influencing the child to rationally consider facts, including his own ethics and welfare, in such a way that disapproved or dangerous drug use is rejected by the child.

It is remarkable in American drug education, and is apparent from a survey of evaluative studies, that the educational efforts are so drug specific. We have seen that De Lone's, Tresan's, and Zinberg et al.s' programs are exceptions. Given the data summarily presented in Chapter 2, it seems clear that children who are at high risk of a drug problem are in that position because of something other than having rationally chosen to flirt with or experience drug catastrophes simply because they were uninformed. Indeed the only study we know which implies an important role of insufficient information or misinformation in the development of extreme drug behavior is that of Chein et al. (1964), whose adolescent pre-addicts were not as aware of the risks of heroin as their neighbors. They were also, of course, different in many other ways. Later observations, for example, those of Feldman (1972), paint a different picture. In this study of street drug users everyone knew about heroin and its dangers. It was the "crazies" who, seeking prestige through their daredevil acceptance of risk, began to "shoot up." This group, too, were different from their peers in many other ways. Their status in seeking adventurism was, we suspect, part of a larger constellation of traits. For heroin users these would probably include strong need for peer approval, poor judgment, some self-destructive tendencies, psychopathy (amorality, exploitativeness, disregard for others), impulsiveness, pleasure seeking, etc. Many psychiatrists and psychologists would join with Pichot *et al.* (1972) to state that those who become extreme drug users are very likely to show and to have had preexisting character or personality disorders.

This knowledge of the relationship, in at least some children, between extreme drug use and other problems in personality and behavior, does provide an alternative or supplement to the rational, cognitive endeavors which characterize most school programs. The alternative approach may take two forms; one is the mental health model and the other is character education. The most intensive example of a (modified) mental health model operating within and as part of a school system is the SPARK program in New York City. We shall describe it and its outcomes later when considering research findings. In other cities the mental health model is not school based, but provides that school authorities serve as case finders. When they identify a child as having a severe drug problem, the child is referred out to a mental health service or professional.

The largest and most emphatic mental health model which stands as an exception to the informational-cognitive specific approach of most schools, is that of the U.S. Office of Education (Office of Education, 1975). This program, devised and implemented by Helen Nowlis, aims to change the ways that teachers and schools think about and deal with children's problems in living. It emphasizes the creation in the school of a helpful, joyful, and constructive child-centered milieu in which teachers and parents join emotionally and intellectually. Drugs are seen as only one of the many experiences posing joys and hazards; the greater the latter the more severe are the child's problems in living. It is the school's task, as a caring environment, to seek to recognize and reduce those problems.

The premises of the program are as follows:

(a) Destructive use of drugs and alcohol is one of a variety of symptoms of underlying problems and pressures which are troubling young people. The strategies that focus on prevention of underlying causes include youth counseling, working with parents, providing alternative satisfactions, educational programs to help students develop skills for coping with loneliness, boredom, alienation, low self-esteem, inadequate abilities in interpersonal communication, problem identification and decision-making.
(b) Simplistic approaches, including complete reliance on information presentation, are rejected. Drug use can arise out of personal problems, family conflict, peer pressure or hazardous social environments.
(c) Schools cannot solve the problem in isolation from their communities.
(d) Each community must make its own problem assessment and identify its own human, cultural and financial resources. The Federal government can provide leadership but success requires local commitment.

(e) The approach of the Office of Education is multiple. It includes leadership training for teachers so teachers are better able to meet the human relations needs of students. It also encompasses personal and family drug counseling support, support for developing programmatic alternatives to drug use, financing community drug awareness workshops, support for teacher training in 1) enhancing communication and social skills, 2) in problem solving, 3) in value clarification, and 4) in setting up parent programs. Support has been given for school-related community efforts such as counseling (peer and professional), drug use surveys, drop-in centers, family counseling and discussion groups, information dissemination centers, interagency coordination, legal aid, improved police-youth relations, juvenile justice diversion programs, law enforcement practice changes, drug law changes, referral programs to other agencies, leadership and counselor training for youth, personally oriented curriculum development, teacher self-awareness development regarding their own drug use and drug values, establishing recreation, crafts, music or meditation activities, community workshops and the like.

There are, as yet, no systematic evaluation data available on the OE effort that describe changes in children's lives or drug use. Administrators and participants offer their impressions, as lessons learned.

Major Lessons Learned and Conclusions Drawn

1. To the extent that a school or any institution:

a) is failing to challenge and to facilitate growth, boredom and either physical or psychological dropping out will occur.
b) is failing to provide opportunities for individual satisfaction and accomplishment, negative self-concept, feelings of failure, unworthiness, and frustration will occur.
c) is failing to respond to legitimate and normal needs, alienation will occur.

All of these negative consequences for youth in failing situations are factors that increase the probability of a variety of personally and socially destructive behavior. If drugs are available and if their use is acceptable to or valued by relevant groups (sub-culture, peer group) the probability is high that this will take the form of destructive use of drugs. Programs that address these needs and promote constructive processes have demonstrated marked reduction in destructive behavior.

2. The problem is not to develop new drug-specific approaches or to train drug-specific preventors; it is rather to select from a variety of approaches judged successful in one or more situations those most appropriate or adaptable as tools to achieve carefully defined objectives designed to solve a carefully defined problem (who is using what substances for what reasons with what results), and

to train those "important others" (teachers, parents, counselors, police, etc.) in skills which can help them perform their functions more effectively.

3. The still widely used traditional reliance on information about drugs, drug effects and the possible personal and social consequences of use of certain drugs has been demonstrated to be ineffective in many cases, counterproductive in some cases. Information is necessary, but only as a tool carefully selected for a specific objective and used with skill. It is not a solution to any problem (note the effect of information about possible risks in smoking, drinking, nutrition, preventive medicine, venereal disease).

4. There exist in most communities and schools the professional, human and financial resources necessary to develop and implement strategies to reduce the occurrence of destructive behavior, including destructive drug and alcohol use. The need is for skills in defining the problem, stating objectives clearly, assessing and mobilizing resources, making institutions more responsive to the needs of young people.

5. Young people themselves must be involved at every step from defining the problem to planning and implementing a response to the problem.

6. Money will not buy the solution to the problem. Caring, commitment, participation and basic human skills are essential.

7. For some students the fostering of healthy personal and social development does reduce destructive behavior, including abuse of drugs and alcohol.

8. Providing leadership training and ongoing technical assistance is more effective than simply funding individual, relatively independent projects without continued and adequate communication with them and through a network of channels among them.

9. A systems approach helps maximize any given effort. Since schools and their related institutions are one of the principle institutions that influence behavior, addressing the total system in which they function is desirable. State Education Agencies, State Boards of Education, teacher education institutions, professional education associations all influence, whether positively or negatively, what a local school district does. In instances where it has been possible to coordinate and enlist the support of all or most of these, local programs tend to be effective and to spread and multiply.

These impressions of thoughtful participants deserve attention. But we must also caution that until hard facts derived from evaluation research are available one will not know which children are assisted by which kind of program, to what extent, in what setting, and at what cost. In the meantime, such programs hold promise for the treatment of individuals for whom drug use is, in fact, symptomatic of personal adjustment difficulties. It also holds promise as a method for asserting standards which can be incorporated, as norms, into peer groups through family, school, community agency, and trained peer influence on these groups.

Of particular importance is the delimited definition of drug behavior to which an Office of Education intervention program is directed. Not "drug abuse," not "problems," not "use," but "destructive use." This focus makes intervention goals clear and outcomes measurable. The definition justifies action under Griffith Edwards' (Judson, 1974) mandate to everyone in the drug business: "The touchstone for all our policies must be *cui bono? For whose good* do we legislate, criminalize, open another clinic, issue another report, mount another television spectacular, lecture to that class of school children. . . . hold to our assumptions? Can the assumed *good* be demonstrated *cui bono?*"

Character Education?

If we define character in terms of certain enduring personality features such as independence, judgment, strength, reliability, high moral development (cf Piaget, 1965), foresightedness, impulse control, and the like, it is evident that most of that youthful drug use which is demonstrably hazardous in terms of health or association with delinquency will be undertaken by those children with what old-fashioned educators would have called, "poor characters." Nowadays "personality maladjustment" might be the term used instead, except that the latter is much broader and, because of that, ought to stand in reduced correlation to the risk of problem drug careers. If it is so, as we believe, that character deficiencies predate the emergence of the problem drug behavior and correlate positively with such behavior in adolescence and later life, one must ask why the school has focused on the limited model of the rational child, instead of on the model of the drug-risk child as deficient in character and in need of character development prior to his or her opportunity to take drugs. Why is it that character education, not only in school but in many families as well, is unfashionable if not distasteful?

Following the work of Piaget, there has been increasing interest in moral development and in its measurement (see Kohlberg, 1966). There has not been a simultaneous increase of interest in American schools in character training. A few studies do give hints that there may, nevertheless, be a role for the schools to play. Erickson (1974), for example, used a special course to move female high school sophomores from the level of conventional to principled morality. Schwilk (1956) demonstrated that elementary school boys could be taught generosity, while Kohlberg (in a set of studies described by Turiel in Mussen *et al.*, (1969) has found it possible to facilitate moral growth, tested in the abstract in teaching situations, as have Hampden and Whitten (1971). Given the fact that problem drug use is most likely to emerge in troubled children and that some of these troubles may be defined characterologically, it seems worth the trouble for schools to learn about possible intervention techniques. If, by training in the early years, there is hope for strengthening character so that children will be able to guide themselves more surely in later years as their opportunities for unsupervised drug use expand, then this would be a worthy undertaking indeed.

William Kay (1975) offers an argument for moral education, one buttressed by research findings and a theoretical exposition. His thesis is that schools must put great emphasis on being places where personal values, individual welfare, and constructive relationships are nourished. This humanistic emphasis does not deny intellectual training but does call for a simultaneous concern for the school as a character-building social system, one closest to the wholesome family in the way all of its members behave and seek to nourish each other. Moral education's long-term goal must be the education of the *next* generation of parents for competence in child rearing. Teachers play a fundamental role, along with the family, as "compassionate authorities"; they provide "disciplined love." Teachers as surrogate parents do this by demonstrating cooperativeness in a classroom milieu which is democratic at the level appropriate to the capacity for moral responsibility which children have.

Kay offers his ideal portrait of a school:

It should be sufficiently large to offer opportunities for the exercise of moral traits and attitudes in work and play and yet be small enough to sustain a community spirit. The process should last from [the age of] three to [the age of] nineteen years, with clearly defined and separate stages. This . . . provides for . . . pastoral oversight [and] . . . for developmentally homogeneous groups . . . The division between school and community [must be] dissolved. During the nursery, primary and middle phases the curricular emphasis could be devoted to refining personal relationships and effective, expressive roles. While the final secondary school could concentrate on academic work, and include studies of the cognitive element of morality. In this way the malevolent influence of disadvantaged homes can be offset and the benevolent influence of privileged homes can be augmented by familiar schools and parental teachers.[b]

To achieve such ends, "teachers should ensure that pupils share in school and classroom organization as much as possible and so participate in a democratic procedure." Teachers are, he argues, responsible for the moral development and the welfare and future of their children even though many wish to disguise how they seek to achieve this, and some try to escape it entirely. With reference to either violence or drugs, these can be, he believes, part of being a "contrapupil" (Barry Sugarman's term), a social role characterizd by immediate pleasures, passivity, autonomy from family, and peer group involvement and loyalty. To eliminate this role, which Kay sees as culturally derived but linked to economic and family inadequacy factors, requires a "radical" remedy, the "transformation of the educational system." The transformation he seeks is not that of Ivan Illich (1971) who would eliminate schools and thus leave families and children in charge (or in anarchy), but the elimination of the impersonal, bureaucratized teaching-machine school and its replacement, insofar as families are not themselves capable and responsible, by the familial and responsible school. One infers from Kay that once a new generation of parents is trained

bKay means by "privileged homes" the greater self-discipline, foresight, and lawfulness which research shows is linked to parental socioeconomic status.

who can be competent parents, parents provided with social resources which enable them to develop moral character in their own offspring, perhaps then the school could be redesigned for primary academic purposes.

Lurking in Kay's humane theme is quite another possibility, an elitist opportunity which he does not intend. If children from wholesome advantaged families are already reasonably assured of eventual moral strength and good character, just as they are reasonably assured of few drug problems, why not let them enjoy intellectual, skill, and interest training to the fullest while only the morally impoverished go to these familial schools? In this two-track system with a vengeance, the already advantaged would emerge not only academically perfected and drug problem free, as they will anyway, but they would be even more assured because the more troubled drug-prone peers would not be present. The impoverished in character might emerge morally improved, and thus safer to live near, but they would be unfit for intellectual vocations. Perhaps, if we are frank about it, that is what happens anyway, except that with present approaches youths impoverished in supporting social resources and in character emerge with neither moral strength nor academic competence.

The Range of Strategies

A range of strategies has been presented or implied. The narrower the conceptual link between children's drug excesses and the model of the rational child, the less change is proposed for the education system. In its most stringent form the principle proposed is that information is a powerful determinant of drug use. That is so because the child uses information to guide his drug deicsions; that is, the child is a rational, self-guiding being. An important modification of this concept occurs when information is held to be powerful, but the response to it is not entirely rational, or at least not as uniform as information providers would wish. Under this modified view no change is proposed for an existing educational system which does not offer drug education, and where drug use levels are low. If it is believed that information serves as a stimulant as well as a guide to decisions, then those children not using drugs but exposed to knowledge about drugs are liable to become aware, interested, and prompted to seek or accept experiences that they would otherwise have rejected. Drug education is then held to be a bad thing. Implicit is the notion that information as such can be dangerous to the naive child who, once informed, seeks drugs, or dangerous to the community which disapproves of that aroused interest regardless of any risk of harm from that drug exploration.

If, on the other hand, it is held that information is not stimulating (or improper), but rather that in its absence a child will use drugs in disapproved or dangerous ways, then all the school need do is to provide information. Under these circumstances information is held to be a uniform good. Confidence in information may be qualified by assumptions about the nature of drug information, its manner and context of presentation, or ages at which the child is deemed to have become a rational decision maker. In any event, under this assumption and for schools which consider it their job to teach facts bearing on issues affecting personal conduct, the only requirement for drug education is that a course be added or modified so that drug information is provided.

At the next stage, if it is believed that facts are not quite enough, but that children need to learn how to use facts in decisions, then decision making must be taught. Until recently this required innovations not in the system as a whole but only in how the drug classes were taught. If it is believed that facts and decisions matter, with personal values also entering in to prejudice what drug choices will be made, then schools must assist in value clarification. This simply adds another feature to the classroom, the opportunity for reflection and discussion, and also perhaps the disguised imposition of teacher morality.

If one moves to the next level, that implied in the mental health or human potentials models, then drug use and problems shift from being central to being either secondary or peripheral. The child's adjustment styles, feelings, ego strength, and interpersonal adequacy are the focus. The school addresses itself to facilitating healthy personal development. Whether or not there is an implicit objective for conduct depends upon the planners. Concern for personal development usually leads to a division into two major paths. In the case of normal children the school seeks to provide a child-centered constructive milieu attentive to emotions and self-esteem. This can be attempted, as in the Office of Education general guideline, through training all school personnel in the importance of interpersonal relations and in using a systems approach to invoke the participation of parents and community resources. Concurrently or alternatively for normal children one can provide intensive maturity-fostering experiences in special nondirective discussion groups (cf Zinberg *et al.*, 1976). Teachers for these groups receive training through the same discussion methods.

For the troubled child special remedial measures must be taken. Counselors, community agencies, and families are to be intensively involved. School personnel as case finders must be trained to identify and attend to troubled children. Referrals and follow-ups are necessary. Within the school special treatment endeavors can be established (cf SPARK: Visco and Finotti, 1974), or transfer of students to alternative schools or other settings may need to be considered.

Should the reformation sought be even broader, as it is for Kay, for whom the central purpose of school is to be altered, moral attainments become more pressing priorities than academic priorities and the whole system is set on its ear. Schools must be redesigned entirely so as to become the "good family" when the genuine family is not good enough. Illich is more radical. He considers the schools to be the entire problem, not the solution, and would close them down completely.

Each of the foregoing models has its appeals, these differing, of course, with the ideology and experience of the viewer. One can predict that the more conventional the school in its information giving stance, the greater its resistance will be to each magnitude of innovation. The fact of resistance does not of course imply that the innovation is thereby worthy. The worth of the intervention model ought to be tested by other than theoretical criteria.

For the research worker, the more limited the concept and the enterprise, the easier it is to observe, both as to a description of the intervention and its actual impact on children's drug use. Yet it may also be, if children's drug use is as complexly determined as the scientific literature suggests, that the more limited the intervention the less chance it has to succeed. Thus within the narrowest activist conception—"drug information will reduce drug risk"—there is also the danger that one is measuring an activity which, at its most productive, can only have a limited effect. At the other extreme, be that school redesign or radical reform, the effects of such a change could be dramatic. That breadth and generality would make it extremely difficult for a research enterprise to say what had really gone on to bring about the changes in drug use that might later be observed.

In our research, reported in later chapters, we have limited ourselves to the test of school programs which are narrowly conceived, conventionally offered, and more easily tested (not that it was easy!). These are the information giving, decision making, and value clarification classroom approaches. Since these are teaching activities which are common and do not require radical innovation, it seemed worthwhile that they be tested for their effects.

Resource Commentaries

We refer the reader to commentaries which bear on the construction curriculum materials as such. An excellent general source of information for resource material and model curricula is the National Clearinghouse for Drug Abuse Information (1970, 72). The U.S. Department of Transportation has developed three noteworthy Alcohol Curriculum Manuals (1973) which cover all school grades. The Girdanos (1972) have published a good drug education handbook for college-age students. Helpful resource material can be found in Imhof (1970), Healy and Manak (1971), Bedworth and D'Elia (1973), and Cornacchia et al. (1973). The reader may also find useful Miller's (1971) description of a student-developed program, the peer group approach of Lawler (1971), and the minimal content outline of Goldstein (1972). There are also other curriculum guides available, e.g., from the American School Health Association and Pharmaceutical Manufacturers Association (1971), Universal Research Systems (1971), the State of Ohio Department of Education and the Educational Research Council of America (1972), and the North Allegheny School District (1971), as well as the Stamford (Conn.) Curriculum Guide (1971).

4 The Evaluation of Drug Education

The considerable materials which propose what drug education ought to do are not matched by an equal volume of information describing what happens in or as a consequence of doing it. While we, in our own work, have sought to offer such data, our research has in turn benefited from the efforts of others. Some of these studies are reviewed in this chapter.

Some of what has been learned by studies in drug education may be anticipated by the more general body of research which constitutes the literature on children's learning. This was well summarized by Stevenson (1972) in a scholarly work that leads to several major conclusions which are good to keep in mind. One conclusion is that children's learning is not easily predicted: the planning of how to teach is not a simple matter. A second conclusion is that common sense expectations may not prove out in practice. A third is that children may learn more from that which was not intended as teaching or "motivated" to be learned than from that which was: "much of children's everyday learning appears to be incidental rather than intentional." A fourth conclusion is that there are many kinds of learning and that children vary in their abilities for each; individual differences are great and make the planning of uniform programs unrealistic. Two sets of characteristics are associated with poor learning. One is low intelligence. The other set are personality traits such as restlessness, tension, short attention span, low aspirations and school work motivation, anxiety, and low self-esteem. Teachers prove to be good raters of proficiency, Stevenson's studies show. Teachers would, we assume, be quite able to sense a correlation between these traits which, as noted in Chapter 2, often characterize high drug risk children and reduce the likelihood of learning. Insofar as drug use problem prevention is directly dependent on the ability to learn in a classroom, one would therefore expect that those children who need most to learn would be the ones least likely to do so. The point is moot of course until there is proof that learning about drugs in the typical didactic setting is related to preventing drug risks.

Among drug education evaluations, there are two areas of work. One focuses on studies of children's attitudes toward drug education, including their use of and preferences for sources of information. The other attends to the impact of education on attitudes, knowledge, emotions, or drug use. In the first area, for example, Smart (1971), using a sample of about 12,000 Canadian students, learned that most children relied on the news media for drug information. This source was more important than friends, family, church, school, and their own experiences combined (we would guess that these Canadian students were not as experienced with illicit drugs as are metropolitan United States students). Drug users (of alcohol, marijuana, LSD, etc.) differed considerably in their information source preferences from nonusers, the former depending more on their own experience and their friends than the latter. Nonusers relied more on school and church than did users. For users, school as a source was described as influential by only 9 percent and for nonusers by only 16 percent; this was in spite of the fact that the survey was conducted during a period when drug education was systematically engaged in by the schools these youngsters were attending.

There are changes linked to age. For children of age six and seven, family loomed large as a source, whereas for late teenagers, peers were most important. After grade 7 school and family become, according to the children's own ratings, inconsequential. With regard to source credibility, Smart's children most trusted the mass media. However, when the older illicit users were singled out, they most trusted not these official and adult sources, but rather their own friends and their own experience. Nonusers trusted scientists and physicians, users did not. Teachers were not particularly trusted, although the researchers felt that teachers could become more credible if trained to meet the children's standards of expertise.

Using a sample of children from a different area, poor Mexican-American as opposed to the predominantly rural Canadian students, the Boyle Heights study in California (Geis et al., 1969) found that students there did not want to be taught by their regular teachers. The California students preferred ex-addicts and physicians as their information sources and also said they preferred discussions over didactic instruction, films, and the like. Drug users and nonusers were the same in these preferences. Some students admitted that films aroused their interest in drug taking. With regard to factual knowledge about drugs, nonusers tended to be either extremely well or poorly informed, and users were moderately informed.

In a Pennsylvania study, Goldstein et al. (1975) asked college students about their high school drug learning. The students reported that they did not have a favorable view of their formal drug education, but preferred the informal situations where they had either read articles or talked with peers to learn about drugs. These students, like those in Canada, thought well of the mass media, those with less drug experience having the higher opinion of newspapers, TV, and radio.

In England, the Institute for the Study of Drug Dependence conducted a wide-ranging educational study with 4880 children ages fourteen to eighteen. In that sample most children at 14 were against drug taking but reasonably knowledgeable and specific in their views. Dorn (1972) reports that these pupils preferred young experts with whom they had long-term access for information; the desire for an informal classroom situation was implied.

In a Chicago survey of 13,000 students, Schaps et al. (1971) found, as in the Canadian study, that nonusers more often relied on school than did users, with the latter getting their information from their friends and their own experience. In all the United States studies, unlike the Canadian, only the nonusers rated the mass media high on credibility. Rating general interest in drug education, Schaps *et al.* report that most students had some interest in learning about drugs, unrelated to age, sex, or drug experience. A Minnesota survey by Cassel and Zander (1974) obtained different results. There, interest in getting drug information dropped as the school grade increased. The range of grades was limited to junior high school.

Schaps and his colleagues asked how drug education programs should be designed. The students strongly held that students themselves should be involved, as Lawler (1971) has done in his programs. Students also wanted experts to assist in program design and did not esteem the programs designed by educators. In Chicago, the older students were more knowledgeable and drug experienced than younger ones, but regardless of "sophistication" students wanted most often to learn about the psychological aspects of drug use, that is, matters of motives, emotions, and mental response. The experts preferred as sources were psychiatrists and psychologists. For physiological information, students wanted to learn from physicians and drug research workers. In exploring the counseling resources students have in mind by asking who could best help them if they had a drug problem, the researcher found a wide range of nominees from which it was concluded there was no recognized counseling resource. School counselors were consistently rejected as helpful because students did not think they would keep private problems confidential, they doubted school counselors' sincerity of interest, and they thought them ignorant. Schaps *et al.* (1971), recognizing the special opportunities the school has to identify drug-troubled youngsters, suggest that a special resource be created to provide individual and group drug counseling.

In another study of Canadian students, Fejer and Smart (1973) found, as had Schaps, that knowledge levels increased with age and grade. So did permissive attitudes toward use, with the qualification that the (academically) better students, who would also be the least involved in drugs, were not so permissive. In this Toronto sample of 4693 students, drug users were the most knowledgeable group and the most permissive. By implication, say Fejer and Smart, if knowledge, permissive attitudes (approval for use and users), and use itself increase together, then one may wonder about the utility of information giving programs, should the goal be the prevention of increased drug use. Lipp *et al.* (1970) raise this same question in their findings, which show that medical students, a group presumably well informed on drugs, have very high rates of use for psychoactive substances.

A Clinical Evaluation

Zinberg *et al.* (1976) have argued that information provision can only further mythology and distortion among children, all of whom are emotionally involved with drug-related issues. In their discussion of evaluation research, they deny the appropriateness, research design, and quantification of outcome measures as such, insisting that clinical study of the process by doing it is the way to understanding. They worked in Massachusetts with 207 students, 7th grade through high school, in seventeen groups, and with 209 teachers in sixteen groups, with fifteen to thirty sessions per group. A predominant theme in children's minds was the question, What's it like to be a grownup? They report that the children were very reluctant to talk to one another. They did not readily let up their guard, for their schools were regimented places where open discussions of feelings and beliefs were not, otherwise, allowed or safe. Discussion of issues relating to social reform, including drugs, precipitates a moral crisis in a group. There were strenuous efforts to insist on structure and on "oughts." They had no alternatives to offer to their current conduct, were cruel and scapegoating to one another, satirized and provoked the teacher, and evaded the substance of their own emotions, conflicts, and ultimate responsibility. Misbehavior increased, for the freedom of the discussion group, at one point, became "freedom to do something you shouldn't." Children and teachers came to the groups "feeling somehow that [students] were bad and wished to be improved," but hating that need because they liked and intended to continue being bad. Moral fervor seemed to buy the right to remain self-indulgent and conventionally immoral. Our inference for drug conduct is that children knew what they were doing was "wrong" and intended to continue doing it. As the meetings went on, the absence of structure and stricture "necessitated the activation of inner morality and constraint." But children and teachers expected a greater personal transformation and were disappointed that it did not occur. At the end, group members had become "more sad than bitter, more mournful than angry, more solicitous than rapacious, more protective than greedy." And for it all, they continued to wonder if they had changed, or had become more moral, to the extent that they were supposed to.

Educational Impact

There are a number of standards by which drug education is evaluated. One set of standards measures how children change (before to after) upon exposure to one or another educational experience. Change can be in knowledge, in attitudes, or in drug use behavior. Properly done, such studies provide for the assignment of children to at least one kind of educational experience and to a control group, with care taken that the two groups are comparable. One should also be sure that the educational experience is what it is supposed to be and that the controls really receive the different noneducational treatment they are supposed to receive. Furthermore, care must be taken in the measurement of change; scales for measuring should have demonstrable reliability and validity and the testing process itself should be free from bias. For example, the teacher should not administer the tests and those scoring them should not know which students were experimental or control subjects.

As one examines the work done so far, one finds that much evaluation is simply commentary unsubstantiated by empirical data. It was to change this state of affairs that the Drug Abuse Council prepared *Accountability in Drug Education* (Abrams *et al.*, 1973), which we recommended in Chapter 1. As for studies based on data, many of these have been surveys which, at best, show changes over time, but, because they have not been designed as experiments, do not allow one to know what accounts for such changes as may emerge. Goodstadt (1974), in a fine review, has detailed many of the methodological problems which exist in both survey and experimental work to date. In consequence, as of 1974, he concluded that there was insufficient scientific evidence from which one could confidently draw conclusions about the effectiveness of drug education. A second conclusion was that the adequate studies to date have shown improvements in knowledge per se, but that efforts to change attitudes and drug use have been ineffective. As we shall see, there are some exceptions to this conclusion. One cannot be sure how it happens that there are inconsistencies from one study to the next, but the most likely explanation is that different kinds of education applied by different people for varying periods of time in different settings, aimed at students with different characteristics and measuring attitude and behavior in different ways, will yield differing results. It is because of such variations that one must be cautious in generalizing from one program, one setting, and one student audience to the next.

One kind of study compares different educational approaches with each other. The (London) Institute for the Study of Drug Dependence work (1974) compared five types of lessons.[a] Over the short term there were differences in effects depending upon the kind of educational effort, but as time passed the differences in effects became less; that is, students who had different educational experiences became more the same. The investigators concluded, however, that "there is a potential for methods to be developed that have different or greater effects" than those they were studying.

Each presentation had some impact on children's outlook, but this was never dramatic. Mild preventive and mild prodrug results happened simultaneously. One outcome measure, reported intentions to use or not use particular drugs, was most immediately affected by the shock film, but these effects passed. The pharmacology film had the greatest long-term effect on reported intentions to use. Another outcome measure, sympathy for drug takers, was most affected immediately by the medical film; over time, all pupils showed

---

[a]The five lesson types were (1) teacher's didactic presentation, (2) "medical" films of bad trips, (3) shock films of injections and a gruesome postmortem, (4) a social history film of a girl becoming an addict and then dying, and (5) a pharmacology film.

more sympathy to users (keep in mind that in this English population few children used drugs illicitly). The investigators saw the general effect of all the films which dealt with people rather than drugs per se as part of a decrease in the otherwise natural tendency to dislike or fear those perceived to be different than oneself. The paradox that the short-term (immediate) and long-term effects (two months later) were different calls attention, methodologically, to the need in drug education evaluation to go beyond one short-impact measure.

The researchers concluded that "no method is likely to have a very decisive, general 'anti-drug' effect," and further that "there is no evidence that an increased anti-drug attitude to 'drugs' in general precludes an increase in intentions to take specific drugs if offered." There was no link between images of the drug taker as such and intentions of specific drug use. This led the researchers to conclude that there can be a number of specific and independent views: "We should not aim at an abstract ideal of 'prevention', but specify the intentions, attitudes and images we consider it most important to modify and how we wish them to change."

Another study comparing one versus another presentation was done by Smart and Fejer (1974). First, reviewing the literature, they found a number of studies showing that persuasions which try to arouse fear had superior results (this is in contrast to some earlier psychological study findings on the results to dental hygiene of high- versus low-fear presentations). The qualification seems to be that this fear-aroused effect can occur best when the information source is trusted. Smart and Fejer, using as a measure changes in the students' statements about their intentions to use marijuana in the future, found that four kinds of fear messages had no special effect on users or nonusers, as compared with no message at all. On the other hand, when instruction was about a drug called MOT (monoamytriptamate), which is nonexistent, all fear instruction had an effect greater than no message. It appears that one short fear-arousing effort makes no difference when the drug is well known to the audience, as in the case of marijuana, but where it is a new (or mythical) compound about which no information is available, then any information, including that presented in a frightening way, can have at least a short-run impact.

There are several studies of the impact of knowledge-transmitting (didactic, factual) teaching. In one, Mason (1972) measured attitude change—without benefit of a control group—and found that among junior high school students a factual program led to increased knowledge, increased curiosity about drugs and their effects, and an increased statement of willingness to use drugs should they themselves feel mental distress. Students also became more liberal with regard to decriminalization of drug use. In another study, Swisher and Warner (1971) found that when they compared traditional classroom teaching to relationship group counseling or to model reinforcement group counseling, the classroom method was as effective in transmitting knowledge. No method changed attitudes or reduced the amount of drug use. Swisher and Hoffman (1971), reviewing other studies, conclude that giving information is likely to be associated with increased use, increased curiosity, and increased liberalization of attitudes. If group counseling incorporates information giving, its results are not appreciably different than other approaches. Stuart (1974), using a Michigan sample of 950 7th and 9th grade pupils, exposed them to factual presentations during a ten-week course. As compared with controls receiving no drug education, students significantly increased their use and sale of marijuana and LSD and their use of alcohol while showing a significant increase in drug information and a decrease in worry about drugs. Stuart found that increases in use occurred most among those students who had both increased knowledge and reduced anxiety, but not among those experiencing only one of these effects. The author warns that there could be an artifact based on an increased willingness of drug education students to admit to use and sales after their coursework, but, excluding that possibility, drug education is found to be counterproductive if the goal is reduction in overall illicit use. If the goal is improved knowledge or reduced worry about drugs, then the drug education program he monitored was successful. A similar finding is reported by Weaver and Tennat (1973) among 452 Texas 8th graders. Both in the short and long term (nine months later), those receiving intensive drug education over three weeks, as compared with controls, increased their knowledge but also increased their drug use.

These results remind one of Joyce's (1973) commentary on the work of Zajonc (1970) which showed, in essence, that repetitive exposure to dehortative information presented in a nonfrightening or nonaversive setting is likely to increase familiarity, interest, and acceptance. Such information program results seen for illicit drugs are also compatible with the lack of success of tobacco smoking education programs. Lieberman Research, Inc., for example (cited in Brecher, 1972), in a study for the American Cancer Society, found that most teenagers recalled anticigarette education in school, most had seen anticigarette messages on TV, and most believed what they had seen and heard to the effect that cigarettes are dangerous. There were only slight differences between smokers and nonsmokers in their recollection of such preventive exposure and in their agreement that heart attack risks were increased by smoking. There was more of a discrepancy between smokers and nonsmokers about cancer (65 percent of the former and 86 percent of the latter agreeing that smoking caused cancer). Clearly, neither the educational experience nor the resulting knowledge had prevented or "cured" smoking by these youngsters. These findings for cigarette use are similar to those for alcohol. Indeed, Brecher (1972) suggests that there may be an increase in the proportion of teenagers recruited to smoking. Dunn (1973), for example, reports that although there had been a drop in the incidence of teenage smoking in the 1960s, presumably in response to educational efforts, there is currently a sharp increase both in the United States and abroad. These findings for cigarettes are similar to those for alcoholism control. The 1973 report of a working group sponsored by the Finnish Foundation for Alcohol Studies and the European Regional Office of WHO concluded:

With alcoholism the practical design of effective preventive policies has proved difficult. There is little evidence that traditional health education can do much to obviate such behavior . . . Patterns of drinking and the origins of abnormal drinking appear to be too deeply rooted in culture and in personality for persuasion or the provision of information to make more than a slight and passing impact. . . .

The results of drug education studies using values as the criteria for change are sometimes positive. Swisher and Piniuk (1974), Swisher and Horman (1974), Swisher and Horan (1974), and Carney (1974) all showed value changes presumably linked to one or another aspect of self-control in drug use. Geis *et al.*'s (1969) report on the Boyle Heights project shows increased caution in attitudes. On the other hand, when the measure of change is behavior in drug use, there are only a few studies with outcomes showing a general preventive effect. Swisher and Piniuk do report that a value clarification approach yielded significant reductions in drug use among secondary school students, as compared with those receiving two other forms of instruction. A Tempe, Arizona program (abstract by Carney, 1974) reports that among 4th, 6th, and 8th graders exposed to value clarification and information approaches, 8th grade boys did show reduced use. Slimmon (1973), reporting preliminarily on a high school project in California using value clarification, found that exposed students had a slower rate of increase in drug use than did controls for particular drugs. Unknown drugs, cocaine, injectable amphetamine, and heroin rates were slowed most.

The most extensive study to date measuring the impact on drug use rates is that of Berberian and Thompson (1974) and Kleber *et al.* (1975) in Connecticut. They surveyed a sample of 4500 junior and senior high school students over three years in twelve towns. Current use of alcohol and illicit substances outside of the home was recorded in a self-report questionnaire. The drug education which children were being given routinely in schools was classified into one of five types (assemblies, regular course work, special courses, and that following two kinds of training for teachers). The students exposed to each were compared. Berberian and Thompson found that "the absence or presence of drug education efforts . . . is not strongly related to changes in drug use rates." When changes were found, they indicated that "drug education efforts are associated with relatively small [i.e., smaller] increases among the three oldest of four age cohorts of students," and, for the younger 7th graders, there were increases in the rate of drug use that were attributable to education. Impact varied with the kind of drug, with no impact shown for amphetamines, barbiturates, cocaine, heroin, and hallucinogens. The type of education also made a difference, with special staff training and regular course work making the most difference. This important study concludes that particular kinds of drug education make a real but minor impact in two directions, reducing the use (i.e., the rate of increase) of some drugs among older students and increasing it for younger ones.

The research report generating the greatest optimism comes from the SPARK program in New York City (Buder, 1973; Visco and Finotti, 1974). Using careful case identification and after-school counseling for students with serious drug problems, it was observed that absenteeism, disciplinary problems, grade averages, and drug-related incidents all changed in a socially desirable way.

The SPARK program incorporates group and individual counseling (especially using trained peers who serve as group leaders), home visits, parent workshops, parent-child group sessions, community involvement, curriculum development, the development of alternative activities to replace drugs, and in-service training for teachers. Its goals are to, "(a) establish a setting within each school where young people can go to learn to like themselves and cope with one another, (b) help students develop the necessary skills to make decisions, solve problems and 'mature,' (c) provide intellectual social, cultural and recreational alternatives to drug abuse, and (d) improve communication with the existing services within each school." The SPARK method involved establishing an intervention and prevention center in some high schools with a drug education specialist, a trained, drug-experienced peer leader, and a professional counselor. Some schools had only a professional drug education specialist. These activities were managed centrally to insure coordination, training, and careful personnel selection for members of the school prevention centers and for drug education specialists. The importance is emphasized of choosing people who are concerned, caring human beings who can deal with their own feelings and understand others, and who are able to benefit from intensive group leadership training. Techniques employed stress role playing of students' interpersonal relations problems, individual counseling, group interaction sessions, parent workshops, referrals of drug emergency cases to the hospital, field trips to drug treatment centers, and student-initiated alternative activities such as poetry, music, karate, yoga, and the like. The SPARK program requires that the school identify self-destructive or trouble-making students, referring them to the SPARK personnel, and it invites referrals from parents, community agencies, and other students and, of course, self-referrals. The cost of maintaining the centers is estimated to be about $100,000 per high school.

The research on SPARK does show dramatic differences. Participants improved while control students became worse on the conduct indices employed as evaluative measures. Although unavoidable, one regrets that the research design did not allow for participating students to be matched on important variables with the controls: participants volunteered for SPARK, controls did not. Therefore, the conclusions about SPARK efficacy must be considered cautiously. This makes it all the more important that SPARK itself be reevaluated using matched or random assignments. It would also be instructive if similar programs were established elsewhere to see what situational factors influence outcome. Roser, for example, (cited in Rubin, 1970) reports a program in Gary, Indiana, where outcome measures similar to those of SPARK were employed, with the exception of drug incidents. There, an experimental group of children who were chronic truants, had poor school attendance, or had serious conduct problems were identified. They were placed in small classes held for half time only and were given tasks which allowed them to feel a sense of success each day. Separate school centers were set up for the program and casework counseling was provided to the parents. It is claimed that truancy disappeared in the group after two years. The report did not describe conduct changes nor did the design utilize a control group. The success reported does suggest that approaches other than those of SPARK, suitable for the setting and the child, are worth trying out. One does suspect that the SPARK approach, like that of the U.S. Office of Education in emphasizing intense and varied trained peer and professional contacts with students, ought to have an impact on lives. Insofar as drug use is symptomatic of youngsters' problems in living, then such relatively massive, individually tailored interventions ought to yield changes in drug habits along with other kinds of conduct. It is one of the advantages of working with children that they do change, do grow, do become more moral, self-disciplined and confident. Education, counseling, or character development usually ought to be successful. Yet this optimistic premise also requires special wariness in research, for it is easy to ascribe to intervention the improvements which might have occurred anyway.

There are some groups of children who are particularly unresponsive, even to continuing professional treatment. Robins (1966) followed up a sample of adults who, as children, had been treated thirty years earlier in a child guidance clinic. The once-neurotic children were leading normal adult lives, but the sociopathic ones, especially those with alcoholic and/or criminal parents, did not respond to treatment. As adults they remained troublesome.

In evaluating children with drug problems who will be educated or treated in or through school, it is important to recognize that there may be several distinct subgroups among those whose superficial behavior—disapproved extreme drug use—appears the same. Some will and some will not respond to one or another change effort. Eventually, one would like to know which children benefit the most from what kind of effort. This is an argument for research, for individually tailored efforts by the school, and for the availability of a variety of intervention modalities.

Limiting ourselves to the information available from rigorously designed scientific evaluations of *all* the forms of drug education, we see that it is too soon to be sure or optimistic. A cautious conclusion is that of Goodstadt's: "There is an almost total lack of evidence in indicating beneficial effects of drug education." For the most part, drug education has induced no behavioral change, although knowledge, and to a lesser extent values and attitudes, are capable of change in the direction desired by educators. Kinder's (1975) brief review offers a similar observation. As Smart and Fejer (1974) comment in their comprehensive monograph, *Drug Education: Current Issues, Future Directions*, ". . . drug education courses of many types can increase knowledge levels, few can change attitudes and one has been shown actually to reduce drug use . . . short educational courses . . . will have no impact on reported drug use."

Actual drug use is resistant to intervention. When one compares different approaches, one does obtain modestly different outcomes, but these may be short term, and definitely appear to depend on the audience, the setting, and the goals of the program. The most common technique, information giving, works if the measure of change is information learning. There is also evidence that as knowledge expands so does tolerance for drug users and for use by the subject himself of some drugs but not of others. As for other methods, recent enthusiasm about value clarification as a teaching method is not accompanied by any richness of proof. Such evidence that exists suggests value clarification changes risk taking and value positions. In three studies, limited by special place and audience, it also reduces the rate of increase in the use of certain illicit drugs. How long that retarding effect lasts is not known nor is it known if the same procedure would work with other students in other settings.

The rule in drug education ought to be to establish realistic and clear goals that are quite specific as to what one wants to accomplish. Then the educator will use a drug education approach which has already been shown to achieve those objectives, testing it while in use to be sure it continues to work while in one's own hands. Yet there are very few educators who require of their teaching the kind of tough evaluation that demonstrates that objectives have been achieved. There are few scientific studies which tell us what programs have worked to date. Remembering the characteristics of high drug risk pupils, and of drug use itself, one sympathizes with how difficult it is for a school to make such of a dent in preventing or reducing problem use. That presentation of facts in drug education has also been demonstrated to increase tolerant attitudes toward drug users and drugs, to expand student curiosity about drugs, and to increase the use of some illicit substances, can also be understood as one considers that familiarity often reduces anxiety and that exposure may enhance interest; children learn that people use drugs because many satisfactions accrue from them.

Summarizing now by type of drug, the data available for tobacco suggest that education (including mass media) has some impact on the recruitment to use cigarettes. What is not clear is why a strong positive impact found five or ten years ago is now not operating, since teenage incidence of use is increasing. This current increase does not mean that those who earlier were inhibited from smoking at what would otherwise have been the age of beginning use (fifteen or sixteen years) have not enjoyed some long-range benefits, even if a new generation of youngsters is now smoking more.[b] Alcoholism prevention efforts in school, as well as efforts to prevent home accidents or traffic accidents, yield rather glum findings. As for the other current illicit drugs, the very limited information available indicates that the use of new or unknown drugs may be retarded by some educational programs as may be the use of injectable substances such as heroin and amphetamines. Yet there is no strong reason to expect school-fostered inhibition of the use of the more popular compounds such as marijuana, LSD, alcohol, or cigarettes. Inhibition can be learned, whether in the form of total abstinence or moderate use; research on family and cultural influences makes that abundantly clear. With few exceptions, that learning of self-restraint has not yet been shown to take place in school.

A Question about Measurement

The foregoing summary statements rely on a large body of data in the tobacco and alcohol field, but on few sound pieces of research in respect to the other illicit drugs. Even with well-designed studies, there are problems of measurement which require that one take all statements of children's drug use rates and measurements of changes in that use as approximations rather than exact figures. Most studies rely on self-reports of what a person says in response to a questionnaire or in an interview about his drug use experience. These self-reports may contain errors (Gaber, 1972). People may exaggerate or lie; they may not know or remember what drugs they have taken, how much, or when; they may misunderstand the wording or meaning of a question; what they say may be misinterpreted by an interviewer or questionnaire coder; or a question may be loaded or biased so as to bring out a particular and misleading reply. Furthermore, people have predilections, varying with background and personality features, which introduce consistent distortions in what they say, as, for example, when there is a tendency to answer with extreme statements, defensive statements, or statements thought to be most socially desirable or pleasing to the teacher or researcher. In consequence, one of the key methodological problems in drug education evaluation is self-report accuracy. It can be compounded if the experience in drug education tends to consistently alter the reply direction of those in a class as opposed, say, to those in a control group. The latter, might, for example, remain more cautious about admitting drug use.

There have been a few studies of measurement error. Boland and Roizen

[b]We have not found follow-up studies which demonstrate that there are critical periods for educational intervention such that, if the onset of use is forestalled during a "normal" or "critical" age, the likelihood of a later recruitment to use is reduced. Such observation, possible by comparison with these several cohorts of smokers (e.g., those achieving the age of ten in 1965 and in 1975), would be very important in planning educational efforts and anticipating "sleeper" effects. Crowdy and Lewthwaite's (1972) findings may hint at such an effect.

(1973) compared the responses of charge account customers at a liquor store to a mailed questionnaire with their purchase records at the store. The researchers found that the sale slips showed fewer purchases than the people reported in their replies, which indicates that these adults were not underreporting, that is, saying they bought less than they did. Schmidt (1973), on the other hand, compared what people said in a family budget survey with observations on their purchasing habits. Here it was found that people did underreport, especially heavy drinkers. Smart and Jackson (cited in Whitehead and Smart, 1972) compared self-reports of marijuana use with the estimates of class representatives, the estimate being the total number with any experience rather than when and how much was used. About 11 percent of the males admitted marijuana use, while 9 percent was the estimate by classmates. In our own research with college students (Blum and Associates, 1969), we used a similar method, comparing self-reports with estimates by our total sample. There we learned that generally the more the drug use the higher and more accurate was the estimate, whereas the greatest estimation errors came from nonusers and infrequent users.

One methodological caution is to ask students whether or not they have used a nonexistent drug. This will yield an estimate of exaggeration of use. Whitehead and Smart (1972) discuss an earlier 1971 survey by Fejer and Smart who found 0.8 percent of the sample saying they had used the fictitious drug MOT. A corroborating pilot study report by Haberman *et al.* (1971) also yielded a figure of less than 1 percent claiming experience with a nonexistent drug. Whitehead and Brook (see Whitehead and Smart, 1972) used the same method but asked about two fictitious drugs on a list of twenty-two drugs. The sample, 106 patients in a drug clinic, reported use at a rate of 7.5 percent. Some of the same patients were given the same set of questions twice, with up to a month or more between inquiries. For all patients and all drugs the rate of agreement (reliability) was 86 percent. Petzel *et al.* (1973) asked high school students about bogus drug use; about 4 percent claimed use. Their characteristics were compared with those not making a false claim; the former were more often male and admitted use of more real drugs as well.

Several studies have examined whether or not anonymity makes a difference to drug use admissions. Luetgert and Armstrong (1973) asked college students to answer marijuana use questions under three conditions. One was an anonymous questionnaire, another a questionnaire marked with a code number, and the third an individual interview. Students were grouped, on the basis of their replies, into four groups ranging from current frequent use to abstinence. More use was reported in the interview than on the questionnaire; anonymity versus coding made no difference on the questionnaire. Harlin (1972) examined the effects of anonymity on children's reports of their cigarette experience and concluded that, on the average, there was no difference in response to smoking questions between 12th graders asked to sign their questionnaires and those asked to submit them anonymously. Cox and Longwell (1974) correlated what

175 heroin addicts in a methadone maintenance program said about their heroin use and what the results of urine testing showed. They found that in 86 percent of the cases there was concurrence (reliability) between the two drug use assessment methods. In a similar study, Ball (cited in Cox and Longwell, 1974) interviewed twenty-five heroin users, also tested by urinalysis. Seventy-two percent of those whose urines showed evidence of opiates admitted to such use during interview. Lest one assume that biological assays such as urine tests are necessarily more accurate than the interviews, let us hasten here to disclaim that. Montalvo et al. (1972) compared urine test results with clinical data which served as the standard (admission by the patient of opiate use on the day of testing, therapist knowledge of patient conduct, and regular records of treat-ment—including methadone, which should show on a urinalysis). The investigators found that only twelve of twenty-four tests that should have shown opiates did so; that is, there was a 50 percent chance that a false negative would have been reported. De Angelis (1972), in a review of biological tests for drugs, analyzes some of the many sources of error that readily occur, noting the frequency of false positives (tests which show that a drug has been used which was not used) and false negatives (assays showing no drug use when one was used).

A different type of validity study proceeded by interviewing a sample of adults who had recently filled a prescription for a psychoactive drug without their knowing that the researchers were aware of their prescriptions. Parry et al. (1971) used this procedure in a midwestern city and found that 72 percent of those filling a sedative prescription admitted to use during the interview, as did 67 percent of those taking stimulants and 83 percent of those taking tranquil-izers. Using two questionnaire forms, one with a color chart showing pictures which included those of the pills they had taken (psychoactive drugs are standardized by size, color, and capsule, depending on the drug and manufac-turer), and the other without the chart, it was found that for tranquilizers there was 71 percent validity without a chart and 83 percent validity with a recognition-prompting chart. The opportunity to recognize a drug one is asked about is seen to reduce inaccuracies (inconsistencies between prescription records and interview statements) from 27 percent to 15 percent. Persons who were inaccurate (invalid or inconsistent responses) tended to be poorly educated (below 8th grade), rated as uncooperative by the interviewer (studies of cooperativeness in medical patients by E. Blum (1958) show this to be a personality variable), male, or did not have English as their mother tongue. From this excellent study we see that drug use measurement errors arise from recollection or understanding failures (i.e., not matching a drug name to what one has taken), and probable defensiveness about the legitimacy (approval) of one versus another kind of drug (greater presumed defensiveness about stimulant use than tranquilizer use). These factors, in turn, are associated with educational background (and possibly, therefore, intelligence and verbal facility), person-ality, sex, and language skills.

Another way of looking at self-report data is to ask people what they intend to do, as for instance to ask about their willingness to use a particular drug, and then to give them a chance to step forward when invited to do so. We (Blum and Ferguson, 1970) used this method on a small sample of male students living in a college dormitory. We arranged, after they completed a check sheet on their willingness to use a number of specific drugs in both a medical experiment and a social situation, that a close friend suggest drug taking to them and then rate them on the basis of this invitation on their social willingness to use the drugs. The association between the friend's rating and the subject's self-rating yielded a high correlation ($r = 0.78$, $p = <0.01$). If this experiment were repeated with females, it is likely that the correlation would not be as high; we found in earlier observations (Blum and Associates, 1964) that women respond to drug taking invitations in terms of their particular relationships to those making the offer. In that same study of dormitory students, we also put two fictitious drugs on the check list. We found no one willing to use these substances socially, but 11 percent were willing to use them in a medical experiment.

Goldstein *et al.* (1974) used a similar method, not in an effort to test immediate validity but as a prediction for drug use developments for Pennsylvania college students. They found that by classifying drugs into eight levels,[c] based on frequency of use and frequency of intent to use, that intentions closely predicted reported developments eight months later. The greatest discrepancy or error was only 8 percent for hard liquor. Goldstein *et al.*'s (1974) estimation technique is, of course, a comparison of one self-report (level used plus intentions) with a later report (level used) and, as such, may be considered a reliability measure. On the other hand, it constitutes one way of predicting later developments in a student population. It provides evidence that most college students either do what they say they have already done or intend to do, or at least consistently say that they have done what they said earlier they were doing or intended to do in regard to drug use.

That paradoxical inference is probably the best that can be said for studies resting on self-reports. It is optimistic in the sense that one does find high levels of consistency which translate into one kind of prediction of drug conduct. Taking the studies reviewed here altogether, we conclude that self-reports are certainly a more practical general survey tool than biological assays, and no more erroneous. The accuracy of self-reports, measured against other possibly dubious standards, is such as to suggest that they can be used to approximate students' levels and kinds of drug use. The least accurate reports, both underreporting and overreporting, will be found among the more extreme users. Even so, their position vis-à-vis more moderate users is detectable through self-reports, al-

---

[c]These levels from most to least prevalent were, in order, tobacco, beer, hard liquor, depressants, cannabis, amphetamines, hallucinogens, and narcotics. It will be seen that a very similar order exists in our younger California sample and led us to make the same grouping in our data. In Goldstein's work and the study we report in this book, the most extreme or unusual drug a student has used defines his classification as a user, i.e., he is a level 1, 2, or 8 user. Kandel's "stages" (1975) represent a similar observation.

though exactness as to their drug conduct cannot be assured. Since we have found no studies on elementary school children, we could not be sure in advance that this fairly reassuring appraisal of drug measurement would apply to our sample.

5

The Research Design and the Drug Use Test: What We Did

This chapter describes the research design for our study of the impact of drug education.[a] It also reports the findings from our examination of the validity and reliability of the self-report form used to measure drug use experience.

Our design required that the drug education effort continue over several years, that it be applied to children of different ages and backgrounds, that it take place in different settings, that it compare several types of educational effort, and that each effort represent the best available in terms of the adequacy of information presented, the quality of materials, and the competence of the teaching staff. Furthermore, it required consistency, to be sure that children in different classrooms received the same educational experience in terms of what was presented. Our definition of success for drug education rested on the demonstration of differential change in children's use of psychoactive drugs. As measured, change was in the rate of increase in the use of several classes of substances. In each instance, educational success through change could be demonstrated only by comparison with a group of like children who did not receive drug education. These definitions required instruments to measure drug use, a research design providing for random assignment of students to control or experimental educational experiences, appropriate data analyses, and the use of statistical inferential methods.

We arranged with schools in four California municipalities to conduct drug education evaluation in their districts. In two cities our sample was drawn from students in the ten elementary schools, three of the schools including 7th and 8th grades. In two other towns we worked in the high schools only, these two high schools being part of a larger regional high school district. We arranged to evaluate the drug education of children initially in the 2nd, 4th, 6th, and 8th grades in the elementary districts. In the high schools we evaluated the students beginning in the 10th grade. Our original intention had been to train and monitor local teachers; this did not work out. To standardize teaching content, style, frequency of contact, and the like, we had to do the teaching ourselves. For this purpose we hired, trained, and supervised well-qualified teachers who became members of our research staff.

The children in our elementary sample in grades 2, 4, and 6 were taught and followed for two and one-half years. In these grades, we began with 271 children

[a]The full technical report of this research contains in greater detail the design, findings, and data analyses. Drug research workers interested in that report, or in the use of the basic data tapes, are invited to write to the author.

in town B, of whom 207 were still enrolled at the end of the two and one-half year period. In the 8th grade, in town B, where our intervention was limited to the one year before graduation and transfer to another district for high school, we began with sixty-three students of whom fifty-six remained in our sample for the full year. In town S, we began in grades 2, 4, and 6, with a total of 956, of whom 767 remained enrolled two and one-half years later. In town S, our 8th grade sample comprised 386 students, of whom 363 remained at the end of our one-year educational period. In the high school in town W, the beginning 10th grade class sample comprised 513 pupils of whom, two years later, 414 were still enrolled. In the other high school in town R, there were 510 enrolled in the 10th grade class of whom 312 remained in our sample at the end of the two-year period.

Our sample size losses were somewhat offset by 209 students who transferred into our participating schools during the course of the study. Our requirements for statistical inclusion in the study for these additional students, as for all others, was the availability of background and performance information in the school file and the students' presence at at least two testing sessions.

As we present our data, it will be seen that the number of students upon whom we report findings is always lower than the total sample upon whom we have data. This occurred because of transfers and dropping out so that there were students who did not complete a sufficient number of drug use tests for some of our analyses, because of scheduling difficulties prohibiting continuation, or because a student's test showed such inconsistency that we were forced to eliminate him or her on the presumption of gross error. We also lost students from our sample when the design protocol could not be followed. Although there were ten inquiries from concerned parents, no students were withdrawn or excused because of parental protest to the teaching program. However, three students in the 2nd and 4th grade cohorts were instructed by their parents to refuse to take part in the drug use tests. In the 6th through 10th grade cohorts, 54 individuals at one time or another refused to complete a test or were otherwise noncooperative. Only one student refused to take any test. Table 5-1 summarizes the composition of the research sample.

The testing program involved two tests yearly, spring and fall. Thus, for the students taught the full two and one-half years there were five self-reports of drug use. One thousand three hundred thirteen students took all five self-report tests. The 8th grade was taught for one full year and followed for two years; the high school classes were taught and tested for a full two years. Present for at least the first and last tests (e.g., tests 1 and 5 or 1 and 4 for the 8th grades and high schools) were 1511 students; 1772 were present at the last test (test 4 or 5) plus at least one of the earlier tests. Our sample size attenuation was considerable but typical for longitudinal experiments with mobile, voluntary populations.

Table 5-1.
Composition of the Research Sample

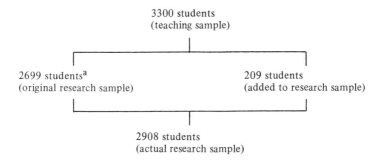

3300 students
(teaching sample)

2699 students[a]
(original research sample)

209 students
(added to research sample)

2908 students
(actual research sample)

[a]The original research sample is considerably less than the teaching sample because of the absence of sufficient information in school folders or because students were members of combination classes not in our designated research classes (e.g., 2nd and 3rd, 3rd and 4th, or 5th and 6th grade combinations). Of this original research sample, 2119 remained at the end of the study, the majority of the loss occurring in grades 8 and 10.

Our Measures

In the 2nd and 4th grade cohorts, through the end of the 4th grade, we used standardized pictures as our drug use test device. Children were individually asked by research staff personnel, who were not their drug education teachers, if they recognized drugs shown in the photographs (these all realistically shown in both still lifes and typical street-use circumstances). If they recognized the substance they were asked for an identification. If the substance was not recognized, no further information was sought by the interviewer. From the 5th grade on, all children replied to written questionnaires, administered in their classrooms and picked up by research staff members. The written questionnaires had been pretested to assure the age appropriateness of the language and clarity of meanings. The questionnaires were later scored and analyzed by others who were not drug education instructors. On the final test additional items were asked. We wanted alternative data to the "Have you ever used . . . ?" inquiry basic to the regular tests, and we wanted a retrospective summary by students as they completed their drug education experience with us. To enhance pupil interest, certain information questions were included that varied upon each subsequent administration. The information items were not scored. Tests were distributed with careful instructions and assurances of complete confidentiality; confidentiality was strictly maintained throughout the study. Only one research person who held the master key list could identify the responses of any named student.

Obtaining Other Information: School Records

In addition to the drug test data provided by the students themselves, we gathered supplementary information from the school records on grades, school problems, school performance, attitudes and interests, parental occupations, family status and problems, health history, and peer relationships. We found that many student files were incomplete and, in consequence, during the data analysis phase, were unable to analyze, as we had proposed to, the relationship of some of these background and performance factors to drug use.

Family Evaluation

For a subsample of students ($N = 225$) drawn on a random sample basis from the 4th, 6th, and 8th grades in the ten elementary schools, we conducted a family study. This substudy was based upon the findings of our earlier work with families (Blum and Associates, 1972a) in which we had found that parental values, child rearing methods, and conduct were highly correlated with children's drug risk. We used an abbreviated family assessment instrument in interviews with the parents in order to establish the family's position on the major variables which we had found predicted drug risk in the earlier study.

Our intention in gathering systematic school and family information was to learn the correlates of one or another sequence of drug use among the youngsters. We wanted to statistically identify clusters or patterns whereby drug use could be seen in connection with a larger picture of family values and school performance and adjustment. That search for patterns constituted one of the basic efforts of our research.

Clinical Observations

In addition to these foregoing major inquiries, we conducted a number of substudies bearing on methodological or clinical issues. A set of family interviews, not related to the test of the drug predictor variables derived from the 1972a (Blum and Associates) study, was conducted by a clinical psychologist and one of our drug teachers. Their goal was to explore in depth how the families felt about drug education and what some of the related attitudinal and value issues might be. The same psychologist sat in on a drug education class in a third nearby high school, one not participating in our major study, and interviewed the students, both immediately and later on, as to their understanding of and reaction to general drug education materials and teaching. The goal was to identify some of the important factors influencing their reactions.

Validity and Reliability of Self-Reports

Another study sought to validate the drug self-reports of children by comparing what students said about their own drug use with what their friends, siblings, and associates said about their drug use. These findings are presented later in this chapter.

Assignment

We designated our control group as the X group, our didactic (information giving) group as Y, and our process education (value clarification, norm setting discussions) as Z. Since children were assigned at random to classes within the individual schools, governed only by a maximal teacher-to-student ratio (which varied by district between twenty and thirty), we were able at the beginning to assign whole classes to one of the three educational modes. Our main constraint was that the fit between our research design requirements and the school organization did not allow assignment to three equal-size groups. Our beginning sample sizes, therefore, were 595 in the X group, 1218 in the Y group, and 991 in the Z group.

There were two basic educational questions addressed in our research: Are there any differences at the end of the two and one-half years (two years in high school, one year in 8th grade) between the controls (X) who had received minimal[b] drug education and those who had received intensive education? Because our Y and Z groups received quite different educations, Y being told the facts without discussion, and Z having value-oriented discussion with very little factual presentation, we also were able to ask the second question: Is information giving superior, inferior, or equal to value clarification and discussion as a drug educational method?

Substudies on Other Influences Within the Educational Experience

Hidden factors can account for the results of experiments. All design efforts in research seek to prevent such false conclusions, usually by procedures such as random assignment of subjects, control groups, and statistical testing, and by substudies of possible other influences. We conducted such substudies, their adequacy limited as sample sizes became smaller. We compared frequency effects

[b]California state law requires all children to receive drug education. We could not therefore have a control group which received none. Our controls were instructed for three class periods a year, receiving some of the basic didactic materials presented to the Y group.

between Y and Z by having one Y subgroup receive the same class frequency as the Z groups; teacher effects were measured by comparing two groups receiving the same education but taught by two different teachers over the full program period; and the effect of class size was compared between half-size (about fourteen students) and full classes. To test for the effects of running varying versus unitary drug education in the same school, we compared schools offering both X and Y with those held to X or Y only. We also asked students if other students in their school were receiving drug education and if so whether theirs was better or worse.

Consumer Satisfaction and Recommendations

At the end of the experiment we asked the students to comment anonymously on the drug education we had given them, including what they thought of their teachers, whether they had learned anything, and what they advised. We also queried the school administrators where we had worked, asking for their criticisms and suggestions. We did not ask a representative sample of parents for their reactions, but we did, as noted, conduct intensive interviews of families whose children were in our experimental program.

Curriculum

Our curriculum presented in detail our Y and Z drug education format. Each lesson plan, theme, resource book, film, or piece of apparatus was described. To ensure uniformity of the presentation of X, Y and Z, each of our teachers met as a group at least once a week to review their work together and each agreed to use the curriculum exactly as drawn. Curriculum development was a team activity. There was greater room for variation in the Z technique, since pupils themselves contributed to the class content through their participation in discussion. Nevertheless, since the same framework was applied theme by theme and step by step in the established sequence of lesson plans, we are confident that the curriculum as drawn up and discussed was the one followed in teaching.

The Self-Report of Drug Use

All of the data bearing on our major questions, "Does drug education have an impact?," "Which kind of education has the most impact and when?," and "What are factors associated with children's drug use?" rest on the self-reported measure.[c]

---

[c]A more detailed presentation of findings on all aspects of this study is to be found in the final report of Grant #DA00097 entitled *Drug Education: Impact and Outlook*, R.H. Blum and Associates, 1975, submitted to the National Institute on Drug Abuse, HEW, Rockville, Md.

We estimated the trustworthiness of the self-report in three ways. One was comparison of information given by the pupil about his own use with estimates of his use made by those in a position to know of his drug conduct (e.g., siblings and close friends). The second was an examination of the consistency of a pupil's reports over time. Since there were five tests from each person (for those who took all tests), each test including exactly the same questions, there were four opportunities to be inconsistent with any one earlier test. A third measure of reliability was to compare the results of a test given in one form (pictures of drugs which a pupil is asked to identify and if identified to say whether or not they had been used) with another form (the questionnaire asking about use of the same drugs).

Our Own Versus Other Estimates of Use

We reasoned that those closest to a student—his friends, siblings, schoolmates, and parents—would be the most likely to be aware of that student's drug use. We therefore enlisted the cooperation of a subset of families randomly chosen from children in grades 4, 6, and 8. Our reliability data are based on information gathered from thirty families with children. Reliability data from the high school sample will be discussed separately.

We first contacted the thirty randomly selected students (called nominators) in the 4th, 6th, and 8th grades, and in a sociometric inquiry asked each to name a maximum of three young people who would fall into each of the following categories: (1) those he liked to spend time with (i.e., friends); (2) those about his own age whom he most admired (i.e., models); and (3) those about his own age whose advice he would follow on drug use (i.e., examples). We also asked the nominator about the drug use of his close friends and for permission to contact his nominees and ask them the same questions that were posed to him. As noted, parental permission was sought and obtained in each case and confidentiality was guaranteed. The nominator's siblings, ten years of age or older, were also interviewed. The sibling interview included questions concerning the estimated drug use of brothers and sisters. Thus we were able to accumulate estimates of the drug use of the thirty student nominators by those we believed were in the best position to know, namely, his friends, peers, and siblings. These reports were subsequently compared with the test answers given by the student nominators in the school testing.

Data analysis reveals that there is greatest agreement between raters and nominators in regard to the rarely used drugs, and that the order is the same for all three grades; there is least agreement on alcohol, then tobacco, and then full agreement, with the exception of 8th grade marijuana, on all other drugs. Raters and nominators fully agree that the nominator is not using the less commonly used substances and disagree more often about the drugs that some nominators say they do use.

The average overall rate of agreement is quite high, 88 percent, and does not differ by more than 1 percent between any three of the class levels, 4, 6, and 8. Agreement varies depending upon the relationship of the rater to the nominee. Across the three classes, sibling estimates most closely agree with nominators, at 91 percent, friends are next, at 84 percent, and examples-models are last, at 81 percent. This is the same order that would describe frequency and intimacy of association among children at these ages. Thus, agreement increases the better the rater knows the subject and spends intimate time with him. That gives us increased confidence in the accuracy of the original self-reports as verified by intimate peer observers.

Another set of comparisons became possible as we went about collecting the reliability data. In order not to reveal to raters that our focus was on the nominating student, each rater (nominee) was presented with a list of five people—four randomly chosen classmates of the nominator plus the original student nominator himself. The nominee rater was asked, "Looking over the list of people, what do you think their general attitude toward smoking (drinking, smoking marijuana, etc.) would be?" "Do you think anyone on the list would smoke? [drink, smoke marijuana, etc.] ?" In this manner, new nominee names reappeared for whom we had both original self-reports of drug use (because the whole class constituted part of our experimental group) as well as estimates from other nominee raters of their drug use. We called these the nominee-classmate sample.

Analysis yields an overall rate of agreement, across cohorts, between drugs and raters, of 80 percent. Agreement is greatest for the illicit drugs, and least for alcohol followed by tobacco. There are only slight differences between kinds of raters, but the trend is for friends to show more agreement with the subject than do classmates (peers) who are not friends. Greatest agreement obtains in the 4th grade cohort and least in the 6th, but the differences are minor. The 4th, 6th, and 8th grade students report more drug use for themselves than their classmates estimate for them. The results suggest that students are not concealing their drug use when they respond to our in-class drug use inquiries.

The High School Reliability Study

Rather than generate what the students termed "paranoia" about our entire program—"What are you asking for anyway, are you a cop?"—we settled for less satisfactory checks. We conducted a reliability study in which we interviewed a randomly selected sample of fifty students, twenty-five from each high school, drawn from our 11th grade classes. The parents of each were asked for permission to see their children in an interview at school. Students were telephoned by a research staff member and offered one dollar to become a member of an "advisory panel" reviewing our instruments. Confidentiality was guaranteed, and every effort was made to generate rapport and interest by the interviewer who was a young, friendly graduate student. After discussing their ideas about the proper role of drug education in the school, the interviewer showed each student a blank copy of the test instrument and asked the student what his replies to each item had been when he had last taken the test in class. He was then asked if, for any reason, any of those replies were inaccurate. If "yes," they were asked what the more accurate reply would be and why the in-class test had been inaccurate.

Comparison of the class test with the interview retest procedure, combining student admissions of inaccuracies, yielded an overall rate of agreement of 89 percent. The greatest disagreements were for alcohol and the barbiturate-amphetamine categories (78 percent agreement), followed by hallucinogens (84 percent agreement), and then heroin-cocaine (92 percent agreement). The greatest agreement was for tobacco, marijuana, and inhalants (all 96 percent). There were no differences in overall rate of agreement between students in the high schools $R1$ and $W1$. This test-retest agreement, under two conditions, is satisfactory. It shows that error does occur in self-reports of drug use, but does not appear to be so great as to negate the use of our regular in-class test instrument.

Our Drug Use Classification Scheme

The basic way in which we describe the drug use of children in the sample is to group them by drug use patterns. We employ two sets of patterns—cross sectional and static—at any one testing time, and longitudinal or types of change over time. We created our patterns much as Goldstein *et al.* (1975) did, ranking drugs by the frequency of reported use (see also Kandel, 1975). A person is classified by the most unusual drug (defined in terms of prevalence rates for the whole sample) whose use he reports. Since the patterns begin with 1 and end at 9, with the most uncommonly used drugs in pattern 9, it can also be said that a person is classified by his level of use.

These ranks are as follows:[d]

Level (pattern) 1. Abstainer: reports no experience in his lifetime with any psychoactive drug used outside of medical care.

Level (pattern) 2. Low-frequency use of the culturally sanctioned substances (nevertheless illegal for youngsters) beer, wine, spirits (liquor), and tobacco: a report of lifetime use of one or more sanctioned substances on no

---

[d]The use (sniffing) of volatile intoxicants such as gasoline, glue, paint thinner, nitrous oxide, hair spray, etc., did not follow, in our sample, the regular and "progressive" scheme (like a Guttman scale), with prevalence increasing with age through grade 11 and with the higher classification also predicting use of all substances in the lower classifications. For that reason, our analysis of volatile intoxicant users is conducted quite separately, and no pattern number is given it.

more than ten occasions or the use of one sanctioned substance on eleven or more occasions.

Level (pattern) 3. High-frequency use of the sanctioned substances beer, wine, spirits, and tobacco: a report of lifetime use on eleven or more occasions of two or more sanctioned substances.

Level (pattern) 4. Low marijuana use: a report of any lifetime use of marijuana with a total frequency of not more than ten occasions.

Level (pattern) 5. High marijuana use: a report of more than ten occasions on which marijuana has been employed.

Level (pattern) 6. Low amphetamine, barbiturate, and hallucinogen use: a report of lifetime use of any amphetamine, barbiturate, or hallucinogen (LSD, STP, mescaline, etc.) with a frequency of not more than ten occasions for any one or a combination of these drugs.

Level (pattern) 7. High amphetamine, barbiturate, and hallucinogen use: a report of more than ten occasions on which any one or a combination of these drugs has been used.

Level (pattern) 8. Low heroin-cocaine use: a report of any lifetime use of heroin-cocaine on not more than ten occasions for any one or for a combination of heroin and cocaine.

Level (pattern) 9. High heroin-cocaine use: a report of more than ten occasions on which any one or combination of these drugs has been used.

The Consistency of Our Classification As A Scale

We used the last test given in each class as a basis to learn how consistent our classification scheme had been in grouping drug use hierarchically, as in the sense of a Guttman scale. All those who were in the "sanctioned drugs only" group had, of course, been abstainers at one time, although by the second grade only 16 percent were still abstainers! Those we classified as marijuana users, who ranked second in prevalence to the most common "sanctioned drugs only" group, had, in 100 percent of the cases, used the sanctioned substances. Thus, in our sample, no youngster reported marijuana use without also reporting alcohol and/or tobacco use. Among those in our next category, the combined amphetamines-barbiturates and hallucinogens, 91 percent reported the use of sanctioned drugs and marijuana. The remaining 9 percent had used sanctioned drugs, but not marijuana. Among those in our most unusual drug category, heroin-cocaine, 77 percent had used all of the other classes of compounds: alcohol-tobacco, marijuana, and amphetamines-barbiturates-hallucinogens.

We handled inhalant users separately from this scaling procedure; that is, we made no assumption of any great regularity in the hierarchical association of inhalant use with other substances. Inhalant users are distributed more broadly over the other categories of use. The modal association, 45 percent, is with sanctioned drug experience only.

Inconsistencies

For all those students who took two or more tests, two kinds of inconsistency were possible. One kind is to report less-frequent drug experience on a later test than on an earlier one; we call this an intensity error. The other inconsistency is to report no use of a drug when, on an earlier test, experience with that drug had been described; that is a substance error. The more tests one has taken, the greater ought to be the opportunity for such errors. There were 406 (31 percent) with one or more inconsistencies. The substance errors, which we deem more serious, are also the more common, with 21 percent of the total sample showing these, whereas 9.8 percent show intensity errors. The inconsistency rate moving from test to test was 8.8 percent, of which approximately 6.3 percent were substance errors and 2.5 percent were intensity errors. About 5 percent of the students were inconsistent on more than one test occasion.

We reasoned that inconsistencies would not be distributed accidentally (by chance, randomly) among all test takers, but instead that there would be greater inconsistencies among (1) students who reported more drug use, and (2) the younger students. We expected the higher-level users (patterns of 6-9, as opposed to the low-use patterns 1-5) to be more inconsistent, because of the personality traits associated with high use, because some might show poor performance during test taking due to acute drug effects, and because the chance for error ought to increase with the reporting of more complex drug behavior. We anticipated that the younger test takers would be inconsistent because of poorer reading and test-taking skills. We did not expect errors to be any greater in any one educational experience group (*X, Y,* or *Z*) as opposed to another.

The rate of inconsistency is higher for the students with the more varied and intense drug experience. Comparing patterns 6-9 and 1-5, this difference was statistically significant ($P \leqslant 0.05$). This effect is uniform for all grade cohorts and all educational experiences, with the one exception of 4th graders in the *X* control group.

With regard to age, we find that the results are partly as expected. Tenth graders do make fewer errors than 6th or 8th graders. The difference is statistically significant. Second and 4th graders, however, make fewer errors (are more consistent) than 6th and 8th graders. Because the youngest children have very limited drug experience—about 97 percent start and end the two and one-half years in patterns 1 (abstainer) and 2 (low sanctioned use)—limited opportunity for making errors exists. These results indicate that among children with varied drug experience, beginning at the 6th grade, the inconsistency error rate is higher than for older youngsters with even more varied drug experience.

For youngsters taking all possible tests, one can calculate the total error rate. This is an inconsistency error at some time (between any two tests) during the course of the study. Using this rate to test for differences among the three educational experience groups, we find a significant difference ($P \leqslant 0.05$) between error rates among the three groups, *X, Y,* and *Z*. The rate is 30.14

percent for X (control), 38.77 percent for Y (didactic), and 30.79 percent for Z (process). This is contrary to our expectations.

Different Kinds of Tests: Visual versus Written

Because we used visual tests in an interview situation for younger students and written (questionnaire) tests for older students, it was necessary to compare the two kinds of instruments for inconsistencies attributable to the differences in testing methods. These would be instrument-related errors in the measurement of drug use. When the changeover from visual to written tests occurred (at the 5th grade level for our 4th grade cohort, $N = 314$), we gave, on the occasion of test 2, the visual test followed at the next class session by the written version. This allowed us to compare drug use as reported at the same time (test 2) by the same children using two different instruments. The results show that there is a significant difference in the drug levels reported in the 5th grade at test 2, depending on whether the instrument is the visual or written. The direction is for greater spread (variation) in drug use patterns on the written form. This includes more extreme drug use levels. We conducted an additional substudy in order to investigate the more conservative use reports on the visual procedure when compared with the written. For a subsample, of thirty-five 4th graders from the 2nd grade cohort and forty-eight 6th graders from the 4th grade cohort, we administered the visual and written forms on the occasion of test 4. In both these cohorts we found confirmation that statistical differences ($P \leqslant 0.05$) obtain between the results on the visual and written forms, with greater spread reported on the written questionnaire. In the 4th and 5th grades, 20 percent and 24 percent of the children gave a different response on one test than on another. In the 6th grade, 29 percent of the children responded differently. The effect of the use of two test forms, visual for the nonreading younger children and written for older children, is that there will be less variety (spread) of drug use reported in the younger group. This bias is not associated with any consistent test-retest error.

Further analyses show that the visual tests are not contributing to any greater between-test error (inconsistency) than is found with written tests.

Comparing Two Different Questionnaire Forms

For seven years (1968-74) San Mateo County, California, the county in which we worked, has conducted an annual drug use survey among the area high schools. Grades 7 and 8 were added to the survey sample in 1969. This county survey (San Mateo County Survey, 1973) was independent of our teaching and drug research inquiries although our intervention years and school samples partly overlapped. We obtained, for comparison purposes, the 1973 county data for grades 7, 8, and 10 in the schools in which we worked. The county survey, using a brief anonymous check list, asked our same 7th, 8th, and 10th grade classes about their drug use during the past twelve months of tobacco, LSD, marijuana, alcoholic beverages (undifferentiated), heroin (asked of high schoolers only), amphetamines, and barbiturates. The county survey was administered within a month of our testing.

Total compatibility in the comparisons was, of course, not possible. Nevertheless, the agreement is high. Tobacco is the exception, perhaps because the lifetime experience question yielded much more use than the county query about use during the last twelve months. Averaging the eighteen measures one obtains an average 3 percent disagreement.

Measuring Declining Use

Our instruments, both visual and written, sought information on both the incidence and prevalence of lifetime drug use. Our premise in evaluating the effects of drug education was that normal childhood development in metropolitan California is characterized by an increasing variety and intensity of drug use (with wide individual variations). Our need, then, was to establish at each testing a baseline of use to see whether or not education would act to restrain further drug use expansion. Thus, our primary measure was to ask, "Have you ever used . . . drug *A, B, C*, etc.?" Nevertheless, for supplemental purposes, we also sought to learn if drug use had declined between one and another testing period.

Summary

In this chapter we have presented data bearing on the adequacy of the child's self-report of drug use. We have compared subjects' reports using our regular instruments with the observations of their drug use made by siblings, friends, and sociometrically nominated drug use models, finding an overall agreement of 88 percent between siblings and subject and 91 percent for 4th, 6th, and 8th graders. On a broader classmate-subject comparison, overall agreement of 80 percent is obtained.

In a high school sample, we compared our drug report with results of an interview which probed for inaccuracies coupled with a retest in a situation where the subject was paid as an "advisor." This test-retest comparison yields agreement of 89 percent. Inconsistencies between and among tests were examined for all students taking the full series of tests, and an overall rate of any error of 31 percent was obtained. This rate varied with individual drug use rates, age, and drug experience, but not with which tests in the series were compared.

For any one test-retest comparison, the visible error (inconsistency) rate was about 9 percent. We then compared our two kinds of tests, visual and written. There was no greater likelihood of inconsistency between a visual and written test, for any given individual taking these, than for that same individual taking one and then another written test at about the same intervals. Overall rates, however, do show that the visual tests yield lower use rates and spreads than do written ones. A final comparison was between a county-administered anonymous check list and our drug report form, although there were important differences in the questions employed by the two instruments. There was about a 12 percent greater reporting of tobacco use when students took our instrument, but differences for all other drug classes were small, 1-2 percent.

All of our estimates of error in our self-report procedure yield similar figures with test-retest comparisons, ranging from 80 to 99 percent agreement, with most at about 89 percent. These figures exclude the higher discrepancy rate found when two forms of the same inquiry, the visual and the written, are compared, for there about 25 percent of the children vary in their reports. The figures also exclude whatever consistent reporting bias may exist in either test-retest or as shared by subjects and peers in the sociometric study. These reliability figures (or validity figures, if one wishes to consider the peer sociometric ratings as the anchor for truth) compare favorably with the studies reported in Chapter 4 and with the standards for reliability generally expected in social science research involving either ratings or self-reports. We conclude, then, that student self-reports contain errors, that these arise from some identifiable sources, but that the reliability and (likely) validity rates are sufficiently high to support the self-report devices which form the basis for our study.

6

Drug Use and the Impact of Drug Education

In this chapter, drug use levels and trends are described, and we offer evidence as to the impact of drug education on them. Measurement of the impact of education is based on a comparison of levels of use in the general groups *X, Y,* and *Z* following exposure to different educational intervention. We expected that normal development for children is to increase the frequency and variety of their drug use, that is, to move upward in the terms of our level of use scheme as they proceed from the 2nd through the 11th grades. Our longitudinal study was limited to a two and one-half year follow-up. Nevertheless, since we observed cohorts[a] of beginning 2nd, 4th, 6th, 8th, and 10th graders for at least two years,[b] we obtained a series of cross sectional measures which, when combined, yield a curve of drug level change for children grades 2 through 11.

Drug Use

The Development of Drug Use Over Time

The graphs in Figure 6-1 display the reported levels of use for each test and for each grade level. For ease of presentation, the figure is divided into four sections, 6-1a-6-1d. They show the test results for each grade on repeat testing along the horizontal—the flow of time. The perpendicular plots increase and decrease in the percentage of children at a given level (pattern). The graphs also note which measures derive from a visual test and which from the written forms.

Figure 6-1 shows that over 80 percent of 2nd graders, by the time of their first drug report, have already had experience with alcoholic beverages or cigarettes, and that marijuana use begins to appear at grade 3, whereas frequent marijuana use (more than ten times) is first reported at grade 6. Illicit pills or injectables—be these amphetamines, barbiturates, or hallucinogens, along with infrequent heroin or cocaine usage—is first reported at grade 5. Frequent heroin-cocaine use (eleven or more occasions) appears first in grade 6 and expands from grade 7 on. The graphs also show that the most unusual drug use

---

[a]A cohort is a specified group followed over time. Thus, our 2nd grade cohort is comprised of all those children whom we began to teach and test in the 2nd grade and whom we followed through to the end of the 4th grade.

[b]Recall we were unable to follow about two-thirds of the 8th graders as they changed districts to go to high schools (9th grade).

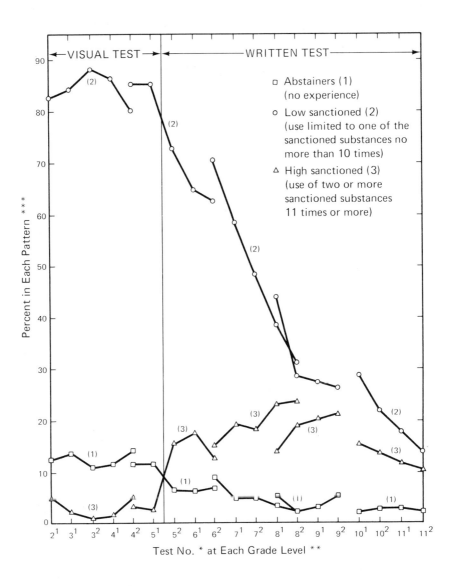

Figure 6-1a. Estimated Prevalence Levels for Abstainers and Sanctioned Usage (Patterns 1, 2, and 3)

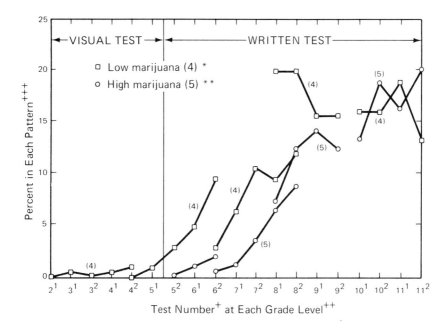

Figure 6-1b. Estimated Prevalence Levels for Marijuana Usage (Patterns 4 and 5)

pattern by the 10th and 11th grades is that of abstinence and that alcohol-tobacco are the most commonly used substances beginning in the 5th grade. By the 8th grade, marijuana use in association with alcohol-tobacco is quite common.

The graphed data support the conclusion that children's drug use expands substantially in both frequency (intensity) and variety between grades 2 and 11. These trends are compatible with the classification scheme which we adopted for categorizing the drug use of children by their highest level of use. Implied in that hierarchy is the assumption that the higher the level beyond level 2, which is the most common one, the less usual is the drug use which it embraces. As noted in Chapter 5, a youngster's classification at a given level presumes the strong

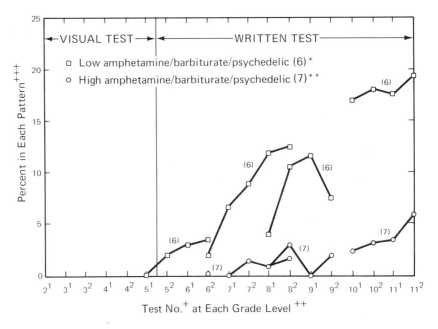

Figure 6-1c. Estimated Prevalence Levels for Amphetamine, Barbiturate, and Psychedelic Usage (Patterns 6 and 7)

likelihood that he will have experienced all of the levels of use lower than his current level.

The Risk of Extreme Use

One would expect that the higher the category of use on an early test then the greater the likelihood that an even higher level of use will be reported as time goes on. To test this expectation, we examined data on students who began in lower levels, 1-5 inclusively, and ended in level 8 or 9. We then compared this proportion with the proportion of students who began in levels 6 and 7 and

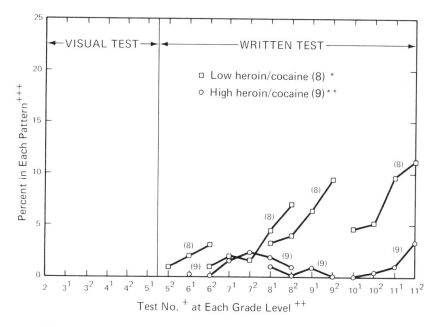

* Low heroin/cocaine—use of either or both substances
  no more than 10 times

** High heroin/cocaine—use of either or both substances
   11 or more times

+ Superscript
++ Base number
+++ Mutually exclusive pattern assignment

Figure 6-1d. Estimated Prevalence Levels for Heroin and Cocaine Usage (Patterns 8 and 9)

ended in level 8 or 9. As expected, termination at an extreme level of drug use is more likely among students initially found to be in a higher rather than in a lower use category. Relevant data appears first for the 6th grade cohort, where the percentage of low-level users becoming high-level users was 9 percent, whereas 50 percent of high-level users ended at extreme levels. In the 8th grade cohort the figures are 3 percent versus 37 percent. For the 10th grade cohort, 7 percent of those initially in low levels became extreme users at the end of the two years, whereas 37 percent of the higher-level students did so. These data also support our concept that classification levels have predictive as well as utilitarian descriptive power. Students with initially high levels of use have an average six times higher risk of becoming extreme users than do lower-level users. These data also suggest, as will be confirmed later, that most youngsters change levels by small increments rather than by great leaps from low to high levels.

An Educational Principle

Normal development is in the direction of ever-widening drug experience. Therefore, insofar as the goals of drug education are to reduce risks associated with higher levels of use, effective preventive intervention will be that which retards the rate of the otherwise expected developmental expansion in drug use frequency and variety.

A Critical Developmental Period?

As we look at graphs a-d in Figure 6-1 we are struck by the changes which occur in the 6th grade cohort, that is, youngsters whom we began to test and teach in the middle of the 6th grade through the 8th grade. During their sojourn in these grades, drug levels 5 (high marijuana) and 9 (high heroin-cocaine) first appear while big leaps are seen to occur at levels 4 (low marijuana), 5 (high marijuana), 6 (low amphetamine-barbiturates and hallucinogens, i.e., the pills), and 8 (low heroin-cocaine). Here, too, the big drop occurs in level 2 (low sanctioned substances) as children move onward and upward through chemicals. The nearest thing to the 6th grade cohort on the graph is the 4th grade cohort. The 4th grade cohort shows a steep rise (when they are in the 5th grade) in level 3 (high liquor-tobacco) and the first appearance of levels 6 and 8. These are, however, limited charges compared with the curves for youngsters in grades 6-8 (our 6th grade cohort). There are stirrings of change by the 5th grade which by the 6th, and then the 7th and 8th, become quite strong. This instability, that is, the great expansion in kinds and intensity of drug use, suggests that in our California setting important events are occurring in children's development and drug conduct beginning at age nine and peaking about ages eleven and twelve. By age thirteen many youngsters have such a broad base of drug experience that it is no surprise if their familiarity and readiness expresses itself in further steady drug use.

By drug class, our data indicate that the most dramatic rise is in liquor use from about ages nine through eleven, from 19 percent to 63 percent. During the same years, cigarette smoking moves from 17 percent to 50 percent with the greatest change in the 6th grade at about age eleven. The earliest use of inhalants (glue, gasoline, aerosols, etc., to be discussed again in Chapter 8) leaps from a zero base in the 4th grade to peak in the 7th, again at about age eleven. A second cluster of drugs involving marijuana, hallucinogens, amphetamines, barbiturates plus cigarettes (which leap from 52 percent to 78 percent) show change as youngsters move from elementary to high school, or grades 8-9, on the average about age fourteen. About 15 percent of all children stay at abstinent or low levels of use (below 3, high-frequency sanctioned drugs). At the other extreme, two-fifths of the entire sample (41 percent are at level 6 or higher (pills, injectables, opiates, cocaine) by the end of the 11th grade.

An Educational Opportunity?

If the 6th grade cohort is going through a critical period in terms of the first burst of expanding psychoactive drugs, then this period also may be particularly important in terms of preventively oriented drug education programs. It might be a time of opportunity, since drug conduct is in a state of flux. That flux may represent an unstable internal or environmental situation for children with respect to those factors which control or determine their use of psychoactive drugs. A different type of opportunity may exist to influence youngsters before they move on to high school. For them, preventive endeavors ought to take place in the 8th grade. If drug education sets as its goal the prevention of the emergence of such risky conduct as experimentation with barbiturates, LSD, inhalants, and injectable heroin and amphetamines, it will have to intervene before rather than after. Our data imply that will have to be, in regions like ours, between the 4th and 9th grade.

With respect to identifying different classroom audiences defined in terms of health and social risks inferred from drug levels, the graphs indicate three clear groups. There are the 15 percent whose drug use continues to be so low through high school that they are unlikely to consume enough of anything to be in a risk group. There are 44 percent who by the end of the 11th grade are frequent users of alcohol and tobacco, some of whom are also regular marijuana smokers. In this group, there will be youngsters who have already experienced alcohol problems; if their lifetime levels remain the same, they will be exposed to further alcohol-related and smoking-induced ill health risks. Some may also be exposed to illicit drug use arrests. Forty-one percent of the sample by the end of grade 11 are at level 6 or higher, embracing users of pills, injectables, opiates, and/or cocaine as well as implying regular alcohol, tobacco, and marijuana use. These two-fifths of our sample do constitute, on the basis of an assumption which extrapolates from level and kind of use to actual risks, a higher-risk sample. While such risks are by no means inevitable, their presence is not to be ignored. One suspects that the school intervention afforded each group should be tailored to fit their situations.

Overall Stability by Grade Cohort

When we discuss changes in pattern levels of drug use we employ two concepts of stability: overall stability and interim stability. Overall stability is the total number of children in a cohort who show no movement from one drug level to another during the total period of our teaching and testing. Instability is overall stability's corollary, the total number showing a change of any kind. Interim stability is a measure of the time-to-instability. In measuring stability, we included only those students with a complete set of tests.

Figure 6-2 below presents a graph of stability data by grade cohort. Inferences from the curves of graphs a-d in Figure 6-1 are substantiated, for the 6th grade cohort shows the least stability of all cohorts, with about 68 percent moving from one level to another during the two and one-half years of the study period. This instability of the 6th graders largely reflects their movement from abstinence to the sanctioned substances, alcohol and tobacco, which use characterizes the adolescent and adult American populations. One might say, then, that in California the time at which children become "adult" in their drug use is in the 6th grade.

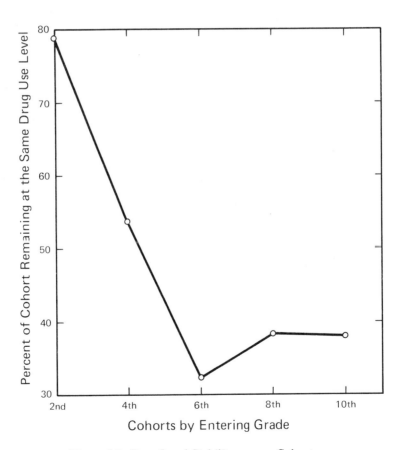

Figure 6-2. Drug Level Stability among Cohorts

The 8th and 10th grade cohorts' instability rates are almost the same (about 39 percent versus 38 percent unstable), but the 8th grade cohort is small here; we lost many 8th graders as they moved into high schools. Had we been able to follow more of them, we suspect that the 8th grade instability would have been shown to be higher. That is in keeping with the curves of graphs b-d in Figure 6-1, where, on illicit unsanctioned substances, we do see drug use changes as youngsters move into the high school setting.

An Educational Comment

Figure 6-2 data are compatible with the argument that if education is to be preventive it should occur before or during age periods where drug use change occurs. This means no later than the 4th and 6th grades for changes which occur in the 6th grade cohort, and no later than the 8th grade for changes which occur with the move to high school in the 9th grade.

When we compare our graphs with recent surveys done elsewhere in the nation (Glenn and Richards, 1974), we find that our California youngsters are precocious. Most other studies are limited to junior and senior high school students, so that the bases for comparison are limited; nevertheless, the prevailing trends through 1974 were for illicit use of unsanctioned substances to be a high school phenomenon. Except for inhalants, which peak by grade 9, substance use increases fairly steadily from grades 7-12 and continues through the early twenties. Some drop in unsanctioned drug use can be expected around age twenty-five, although alcohol and tobacco intensity can continue to increase in later years. To the extent that these other studies do not underreport elementary school drug use, then in other communities preventive drug education may be considered for somewhat older grades than would be required in California. If the trends described in Chapter 2 continue, the use of psychoactive drugs will become more prevalent elsewhere in lower grade levels.

The Impact of Drug Education

Does Education Make A Difference?

From the standpoint of our statistical analyses, there are two general criteria we use in testing our data to learn whether one form of drug education has a different impact on children's drug use than does another. Keep in mind that we have three forms of education: didactic, process, and the minimally exposed control group. One way to look for an education effect is to look at the stability of drug use. Stability in general is defined as no change in drug use from one test to another. Use is defined in terms of our classification scheme of pattern levels. We distinguish two kinds of stability: interim or short-term stability when no change occurs in drug levels between any two tests excluding the very first and very last test; and overall stability defined as no change occurring in drug use levels during the course of the study as measured by comparing the first and last tests. (Anyone going up and then going down on interim measures was inconsistent because our question on use was, "Have you ever . . . ?") Instability, as the opposite of stability, occurs whenever any (consistent) change occurs, be that on interim measures or on the beginning-to-end measure.

A second way to look at educational impact is to look at spread. Spread refers to the degree or extent of change which takes place among those students whose levels of use are unstable. Change is defined in terms of the drug use pattern levels in our classification scheme.

There are, in turn, several ways by which one can examine an individual's spread of drug use over time. We chose to examine these changes in relationship to what others in a student's cohort did, comparing to see if an individual's changes in drug use were like those of the majority, were uncommon, or were so unusual that they could be termed "extreme." These characterizations form the basis for our definitions of patterns of drug use change over time, a classification system which we used in identifying the correlates of change. We considered as "extreme" the 10 percent of the total sample in any given starting level for each cohort whose change patterns showed the largest shift. Thus, if 200 students in a cohort started at level 2 and two and one-half years later there were 20 of those students at levels 7, 8, and 9, this large shifting unusual group of 10 percent would be our extremes for that cohort and starting level. Their spread or extent of shifting is greater than the more common patterns, which would have been from beginning level 2 to ending levels 2-6. The most common consistent changes are low-order spreads, e.g., from level 2 to 3, whereas those sample members in the extreme group, approximately 10 percent will show the most dramatic spread of use across levels, e.g., from level 2 to level 7, 8, or 9.

The second criterion to be used for assessing whether or not drug education has an effect on student usage is measured in terms of the percentage of students reporting an extreme (10 percent of total cohort population) shift from their initial starting level. Because most of the students initially started at level 2, all comparisons were made with respect to this subset. For comparability when the groups had different stability values we computed the conditional extremes.[c]

In summary, we measured educational impact by observing whether exposure to different educational experiences, X, Y, or Z led to differences among X Y, or Z students' drug use over time. We created a classification scheme for measuring drug use at any one point in time and we created a scheme for describing drug use over time in terms of patterns. Stable patterns were those

---

[c]As a convenience in data analysis, we calculated "conditional extremes." This ratio was obtained by dividing the observed number of extreme students by the number of unstable students. This analysis considered only cases where students started at level 2. This figure gives us a percentage for extreme changes. "Conditional extremes" can be directly compared among groups even though groups had dissimilar fractions of overall stability.

where there was no change in levels from beginning to ending tests. Unstable patterns were those where there was change, drug use moving from a lower to a higher level over time. The distribution of these patterns of change from lower to higher levels for a cohort is the spread. Cohorts are described empirically in terms of the stable, common, and extreme patterns. Extreme is defined as comprising the patterns that characterize the most unusual 10 percent of any cohort.

If we observe that one form of drug education is associated with greater stability, then we can conclude that the educational intervention is more effective as compared with others where there is greater instability. Likewise, if we observe that one form of drug education, as compared with others, is associated with lesser spread, i.e., a smaller percentage of conditional extremes, then we can conclude that such educational intervention is more effective. Judgments as to impact and effectiveness here are always in terms of the comparison of the *X, Y,* and *Z* groups, of lesser versus greater stability, and/or of lesser versus greater spread.

Before any test of differences in spread can be made, one must be sure that each of the three different educational experience groups, *X, Y,* and *Z*, started, on the average, at the same level. If, for example, some biasing effect had occurred in the assignment of students to groups *X, Y,* or *Z*, so that the majority, say in *X*, started at level 1 in a given cohort, whereas the majority in *Y* started at level 4, then our spread measure would be meaningless. Recall that our design sought to assure a random assignment of students to each group. Randomizing procedures ordinarily distribute people in such a way that no one group differs from another in the characteristics which must be controlled. When we array our starting patterns for cohorts 2-8, we find that they are not significantly different. We note, however, that in the 10th grade there were markedly more low marijuana users, level 4, in the *X* group than in the *Z* group, and vice versa for the high marijuana users, level 5. We do not find evidence of any selection bias to account for this.

*The Impact of Drug Education: Negative Findings on
Interim Stability*

One possible effect of drug education is on interim stability. If one looks at all students moving from one level of use to another during the course of our teaching, one wonders if those exposed to one educational experience waited longer before shifting than did those in the control group. Put another way, one asks if there are differences among the educational groups in the time when those drug use changes which did occur were first observed.

We examined all cohorts for the time of first change during the period of teaching and testing. There were no statistically significant differences among the X, Y, and Z groups. With no evidence of an educational impact on interim stability, we conclude that there is no short-term effect which delays the onset of drug use change.

Overall Stability Undistinguished by Cohort
and Starting Level

Overall stability is the percentage of students that did not change their drug level during the full period of our teaching and observation. To make this measure our population was restricted to those students completing both the first and last tests given to each cohort, regardless of interim test omissions. Stated as a general hypothesis, the question of educational impact asks if students who received minimal drug education, the controls, were less stable (had a higher proportion moving from a lower to a higher drug use level) than were students in the didactic Y, or process Z educational groups. One would assume, of course, that if education "worked" such a difference would obtain.

Our initial test of the data combined all cohorts and students regardless of their starting levels. Analysis reveals that, using this crude combinatorial approach, that there are no statistically significant ($P > 0.05$) differences between X as opposed to Y or Z, nor between Y and Z.

The Impact of Drug Education: Positive
Findings on Stability and Spread

In order to examine our data cohort by cohort and to improve the basis for statistical testing by limiting analysis to those groups (levels) of sufficient sample size, a more refined procedure was used. It restricted itself to within-cohort testing and to those students who began at level 2, in which a majority of the overall population fell and which was also the modal category for every cohort.

Figure 6-3a and 6-3b charts the results. Figure 6-3a shows that the control mode X, yields a higher percentage of students that remain stable over time for all cohorts. Of the two intensive interventions, the didactic mode, Y, yields the least stability for all grade levels, and, by that criterion of impact, is least preferred over X and Z. The process mode, Z, is consistently in a middle position.

The shapes of the mode curves with grade levels (Figure 6-3a) are similar, starting with high percentages (70 percent) at the 4th grade level then tending to level off during the 6th through the 10th grades. The control mode levels off at about 55 percent, while the process and didactic modes level off just above 30 percent. Thus, there is over a 20 percent difference between the most stable, X, and the least stable, Z, groups.

Figure 6-3b indicates the distribution of (conditional) extreme shifts among the three different educational experience groups. Here, too, the controls, X,

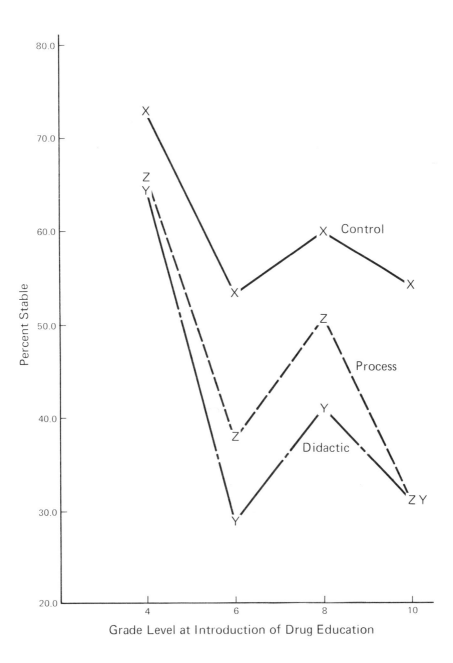

Figure 6-3a. Estimated Percentage of Cohorts that Remain Stable within Drug Pattern (2) Over a Two-year Period, All Students Starting from Pattern (2)

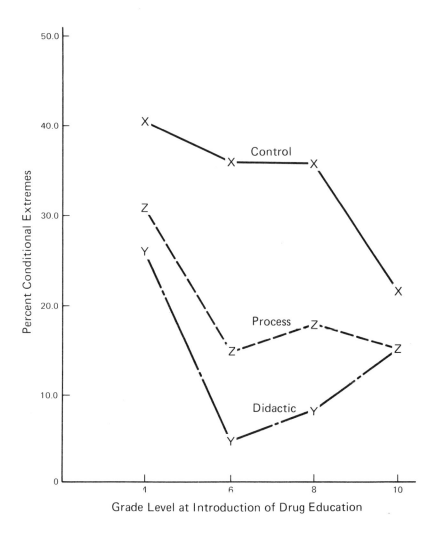

Figure 6-3b. Estimated Percentage of Nonstable Cohorts Reporting Extreme Pattern Change (10% Criterion) Over a Two-year Period, All Students Starting from Pattern (2)

stand apart from the educational groups Y and Z over all cohorts. In this case, with extreme change least preferred, the control is associated with the least-preferred outcome. The didactic, on the other hand, is consistently observed to yield the least-extreme spread of change and, using the spread criteria, is most preferred. Process maintains a middle position. The shape of the control curve differs from those of the experimental educational interventions; the former is convex, and the latter two are concave. This focuses our attention on the region of greatest disparity between the control and both the process and didactic groups, which is in the 6th and 8th grade cohorts. For the 6th grade cohort the percentage of conditional extremes is less than 5 percent among didactic students and almost 40 percent among control students.

The control mode maintains more students in a stable drug use condition over time but simultaneously yields more extreme changes among those students who do make shifts, that is, who show instability in drug use levels. The didactic intervention does not do well if the goal is to maintain stability, i.e., to prevent any change, but it does best when the goal is to prevent extreme shifts upward in drug use levels among students who do increase the intensity or variety of their psychoactive drug use. The process approach is consistently in the middle, yielding more stability than the didactic mode and less extreme spread of change than the control mode. These effects are most visible for the 6th grade cohort, diminished for the 8th grade cohort, less noticeable in the 4th grade cohort, and minor, indeed, for the 10th grade cohort. Interpretation of impact is restricted by lack of knowledge on effects longer than two and one-half years. We are also unable to say, given our earlier demonstration that differences between X, Y, and Z were small when interim stability was examined, what a minimum education period might have to be in order to show an impact. Indeed, it is possible that the two or two and one-half year period may be the shortest effective intervention.

The Optimal Age for Drug Education

Figure 6-4a and 6-4b shows that the greatest difference between educational modes, as measured by the percentage of students affected, appears to be in the 6th grade cohort. Only at the 6th grade level are statistically significant differences obtained. One cannot exclude the likelihood that had sample sizes been larger at the other grade levels, e.g., at grade level 8, significant differences would also have been found.

Figure 6-4b indicates the relative advantages of the didactic and process modes over the control mode when using the criterion of conditional extremes. Such advantages rise and then fall after reaching a peak at the 6th grade level. Differences are statistically significant at the 6th grade level.

Consistency of Results

When the effects of three educational experiences over cohorts are ranked for stability and spread and a nonparametric test is made, one finds that there is less than a 3 percent chance that the consistency observed would occur as a result of random fluctuation (i.e., $P \leqslant 0.03$). We conclude not only that

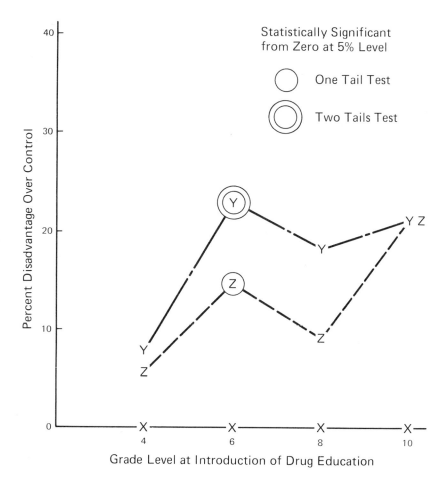

Figure 6-4a. Estimated Percentage Disadvantage of the Didactic (*Y*) and Process (*Z*) Modes over the Control (*X*) Based on the Criterion of Maintaining Stability

educational mode affects stability and spread at the 6th grade cohort level, but that the same trend exists for the 4th and 8th grade cohorts.

Hidden Influences

The research design sought to control for influences other than drug education, influences which may have accounted for the results of the comparison of the *X*,

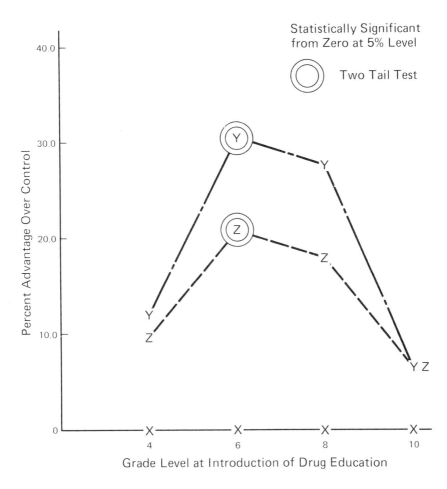

Figure 6-4b. Estimated Percentage Advantage of the Didactic (*Y*) and Process (*Z*) Modes over the Control (*X*) Based on Criterion of Conditional Extremes

Y, and *Z* educational experiences. The possible influences under study were class size, class frequency, teacher, school differences in terms of neighborhood income levels, diverse versus homogeneous drug education programs within the school, and, in relation to this, children's awareness of other kinds of drug education being offered in their school.

Since our major commitment was to testing the impact of education under routine school conditions, and since each such design control required that unusual subgroups be set up, these inquiries depended on smaller samples. During the course of the study, administrative problems arose such that these samples were attenuated. Therefore, our examination of possible hidden influences is less conclusive than we would have wished. We were aware that such influences, if operating, could interact with our teaching intervention (our independent variable), the detection of which would require additional controls and tests for interaction. Unfortunately, such interaction studies were not feasible.

To test for the influence of class size, we compared small versus ordinary-size process education classes. We found no significant difference in educational impact as a function of class size. To test for the influence of class frequency, we taught one set of didactic, Y, classes with the same frequency as the process classes, which met twice as often as the regular Y classes. We found no differences between the more- and less-frequent Y classes in their final drug use levels. To test for teacher effects, we compared one cohort within the same mode and school. One set of students had one teacher for the full two and one-half years, another set had another. There were no differences in educational impact. Each of these conclusions is tentative and requires verification through further research. For the present we may only say that, within the limits of our design, class size for process education, frequency for didactic education, or teacher for process education, do not appear to account for the differences we have observed between process and didactic education. We suggest that those differences are attributable to the difference in the educational style itself. The control, X group differed radically from Y and Z in class frequency, but not in class size or in teachers doing the work. It is reasonable to expect that major differences in exposure to drug education deserve further investigation.[d]

The test for interaction effects was limited to the socioeconomic status, measured by census tract data, from which the populations of the schools were drawn. A statistically significant difference is found in beginning drug use levels, depending upon the socioeconomic status of school populations; higher-income elementary schools seem to have higher beginning drug use levels. No interaction between a school population's income status and the impact of drug education was found. Nor is any significant between-school difference observed when the variable is homogeneity versus diversity of drug education programs within a school. Further examination of the homogeneity-diversity variable, based on youngsters' awareness of whether they were getting the same education as others in their school, provides no evidence that control group students were more aware of or felt they were receiving poorer drug education, as compared with Y

[d]In a set of major studies Inkeles (1975) and his colleagues have been studying the influences which account for people in underdeveloped countries having "modern" views. (In this sense, drug experimenters might be called "modern.") They find that the duration of time spent in school was one of the most significant influences. Duration was more important than kind of school in shaping attitudes.

or *Z* students. And *Y* and *Z* students do not differentially feel discriminated against by virtue of the kind of drug education they are receiving. We conclude that the differences between *X* and *Y* or *Z* education are not attributable to controls being aware of or feeling that they are receiving less-adequate drug education. With regard to the study of other interaction effects, as well as further clarification of the role of class frequency, class size, or teacher impact on the efficacy of drug education, further research is in order.

Cautions, Questions, Comments for Educators

The observations and interpretations offered in this chapter are restricted. We do not know about any decline in drug use among individuals which may be attributable to drug education, declines which could counter the developmental trend of increasing drug use during elementary and high school years in California. We do not know what long-term effects, if any, may occur in consequence of the drug education we have given. We cannot be certain that the differences between *X, Y,* and *Z* students which we have observed are attributable to what we say we did. We attempted to test for the influence of the obvious possible extraneous influences—classroom size, frequency of presentation, teacher differences, school milieu—and we trained our teachers to follow the same curriculum. Yet we must ask, What didn't we think about that may have led to these differences? What did we try to control but fail to control?

There are some questions raised which bear on educational policy. They focus on long-range effects. One question asks, Is there not a possibility that the effects of educational impact in the long run will not be the same after all? This would occur if a student who is moderately stimulated through drug education to increase his drug use (as in the *Y* and *Z* groups), but who is simultaneously restrained by *Y* and *Z* education in the extent of his spread of use, ends up (if he receives no further drug education) at age twenty or twenty-five at the same place as the minimally educated control group member whose drug spread is delayed, but when it occurs expands rapidly.

Behind this question there lurks the issue of critical periods. For example, if a development does not occur when the child is at the stage when it ordinarily occurs, will that same development be less likely to occur in some future and "less-ready" stage? This question, in turn, could hinge on biological as well as environmental factors. We have not seen any studies which bear directly on this issue of critical periods in human drug use development, except for that work which describes the ill effects on infants of drugs taken in pregnancy (Brazelton, 1970). One does know (U.S. Department of HEW, Public Health Service, 1973) that people who begin smoking earlier are more likely than late beginners to continue to smoke. It is also the case (Jellinek, 1960) that children who are early introduced to alcohol and drink it routinely instead of other beverages (as in

France) develop alcoholism. In our own work (Blum and Associates, 1972a) we found that the more-involved drug users had earlier illicit experiences.

On the basis of such findings, one could predict that drug education which manages to delay the onset of regular use of substances can have enduring effects. In that case, the preventive strategy would be to control spread rather than stability. This assumes that there exists that as yet undemonstrated critical intervention period.

The alternative possibility that the stability enjoyed by the control group is only temporary is easily entertained. Many studies show peer-influenced drug use expansion, as, for example, upon entrance to high school. If early intervention does not have a long-lasting "immunizing" effect, then one would have to design some effective continuing educational intervention to counteract that later peer influence, unless, of course, effective early intervention had been so widespread that a major shift in drug use occurs. In such an unlikely instance, the peer majority in high school or college would be more abstinent than is currently the case. If the argument for no long-lasting early education effect is correct, then any intervention early or late is a waste of time and money.

It could also be argued that given no long-term effect, any early intervention would be disadvantageous if it had the effects we demonstrated. That would occur if the only rule operating was one of those we observed, that the higher the initial level of use during a developmentally drug-expansive period, the higher the level at a later time. Because education is destabilizing—stimulating—initial levels are raised. Yet our data on spread suggest that some kind of self-limiting feature is associated with education. Perhaps these constraints are similar to ones which account for abstinence or low-level use among most youngsters when they are exposed to high-use peers. Perhaps the constraints are tied to those which emerge with age to slow or reverse formerly high levels of use. No one knows, but these questions of the duration of positive early intervention effects, possibly in connection with critical stages and the reinforcement of self-limiting features, are powerfully important for educational policy as well as for research on children's drug use.

The choice of minimal or no education versus process education, versus didactic education is not necessarily between one extreme, no education, versus the other, didactic education. One could elect the moderate course instead, arguing that with the limited knowledge available the best bet would be to employ the process mode, which has some positive impact both in stabilizing drug use—although not as much as minimal education—and in restraining extremism in use—although not as much as the didactic mode. This is a defensible compromise. Alternatively, one might separate audiences, for instance, dividing elementary school children into two groups. One could assign the students with characteristics most likely to make them candidates for early and rapid drug use expansion to classes that do not aim at stability—which would be too much to hope for—but rather at moderating or channeling drug interest expression: they would experience the didactic method. For children whose characteristics indicate that their ordinary development would not involve much drug experimentation, there would be no drug education at all.

In spite of our initially large sample, many of the subgroups turned out to be small. In consequence, we limited the impact analyses to our largest group, those students found on the first test to be at level 2. As a result, we can make no statements about what happens in elementary school drug education to students in the unanalyzed, less-common starting categories. It would be heartening to believe that they were the same as our level 2 sample, but there is no evidence for believing one way or the other. A strong limitation is, therefore, placed upon our findings. It will take another study using many more students before we know how drug education affects those whose first educational experience finds them at higher use levels. Our guess is that these higher-level users, whom we know are at risk of expansion to even higher levels, are, in fact, more like the older 10th graders whom our study found to be unresponsive to drug education in any form.

As we speak of 20-35 percent of a student population whose drug use is affected because they experience one form of education rather than another, one should not forget the 65-80 percent for whom the educational impact is nil. The size of that majority of students becomes greater with age, so that by the 10th grade one can say that no student has been responsive to any form of drug education, be it intensive or minimal. To illustrate the extreme, consider the ten students (0.3 percent of the sample) who jumped from abstinence to heroin-cocaine in the course of our study, and look at the 11 percent of our 10th grade cohort who became users of heroin and/or cocaine while we were teaching them. Or look at the 23 percent of that cohort who moved into level 6, or higher to the pills and injectables, while they were experiencing our ministrations. Our optimistic generalizations cannot ignore our failure to influence the majority or to stop leaps into extreme drug use in the teenage sector of our sample.

Keep in mind, as well, that one does not know the relationship between prevalence of higher levels of drug use and the incidence of actual difficulties in students' lives. The "risk" of moving into a higher-level group is by no means the same thing as the "risk" of actually getting sick, arrested, addicted, or otherwise fouled up. Uncertainty about the rates for demonstrable ill effects leads to the question, "If we don't know the extent of real risk, is any drug education worth the trouble?" So stated, it is no longer a question of choosing alternatives within drug education but a question of any drug education at all. This is a policy issue. "Worth" is a matter of dollars and cents. Teaching and administrative time is not free. Worth is also a matter of values and choices. The student spending twenty hours a year in drug education is deprived of the chance of spending twenty hours a year learning something else. And worth is a matter of balancing nonequivalents. Is it worthwhile, hypothetically, to "prevent," during one year, four cases of needle-induced hepatitis, three drunken automobile accidents, two psychiatric admissions, and one inhalant-induced death in a population of 3000 children when the cost of their drug education is $30,000? We do not know, in fact, if our effort prevented any such incidents. We do know that our drug education program cost about $30 per student per year. A program integrated into a school system should, however, cost much less.

Summary

The three educational modes did have different effects on the progression of students from one drug level to another over the several years of our teaching. The effect is most pronounced for the 6th grade cohort, which received drug education during the 6th, 7th, and 8th grades. Educational impact is also present through the 4th and 5th and into the 9th grades. There are two kinds of educational impact. One is destabilizing: more children move to higher levels of drug use as they experience our intervention. Stability, on the other hand, is most pronounced for those with the least drug education, the control group. The other change is the extent of spread. Expansion in drug use intensity and variety among those students showing any change in levels of use is most restrained among those experiencing didactic education, moderately restrained among process-educated students, and most extreme among the control group. About 25 percent of the didactic group will be "destabilized" by drug education in comparison with more-stable controls, whereas over 30 percent more controls than didactic students are likely to make extreme leaps in their drug use levels once they do begin to change.

7

Predicting Stability and Change

In this chapter, personal, school, and family characteristics associated with patterns of drug use development are described. These are features helpful in predicting which students will show which kinds of drug use over time. The conditions of data gathering and analysis limit us to tentative generalizations.

School Characteristics

For all students, we sought from school records information on their persons, their background, and their school performance. In addition, we conducted an end-of-study interview with school administrators and teachers to identify students who offered or had special problems. There were thirty-eight characteristics on which data was sometime available, as shown in Table 7-1.

Another step was the construction of a classification system for categorizing drug use changes over the period of our teaching and testing. This scheme describes, for each beginning drug level within each cohort, three possible change patterns from the first to the last test. One is a stable pattern, with no change in levels. The second is the most common change, empirically determined and embracing all students, and shows a change in drug use levels, except for the approximate 10 percent showing the most extreme changes. As noted in Chapter 6, the extreme changes were the students who showed the greatest spread, moving from low to high levels of use. Since there were nine possible beginning levels according to our initial scheme, and three change patterns for each level, each cohort could be categorized, theoretically, into twenty-seven patterns. In reality, the distribution in each cohort was less than twenty-seven patterns, with the fewest patterns occurring in the youngest 2nd grade cohort (that showing least variability and change) and the most patterns occurring in the oldest 10th grade cohort.

The third procedure was the selection of a statistical test and the development of a computer program suitable for description of and inference from the data. We employed a multiple discriminant analysis. This method requires that sample sizes be large, no group less than $N = 50$ for stable, common, and extreme combined. The product of the calculations is a ranking of variables (student characteristics) in terms of the power each has to discriminate among the several groups considered. By this means, one is able to state not only how the stable students differed from common and extreme, or common differed

Table 7-1.
Sources for Student Characteristics

Characteristic	Source				
	Clerical records	Teacher rating	Computer printout	Administrative comments	Teacher evaluation
Sex	X				
Ethnic background	X				
Father's occupation	X				
Mother's occupation	X				
Number of siblings	X				
Family status	X	X			
Domicile status	X	X			
Report card history					
grades	X				
trend	X				
Interests and activities					
arts		X			
crafts		X			
outdoor		X			
indoor		X			
general participant		X			
Leadership		X		X	
Attitudes toward self		X		X	
Relationship with peers		X		X	
Feelings about school		X		X	
Family/home relationship		X		X	
Behavior problems	X	X		X	
Attendance problems	X	X	X	X	
Suspected drug use	X	X		X	
Referral to agencies					
(negative)	X	X		X	
Confidential file	X				
Physical fitness test	X				
Excessive absences	X			X	
Excessive transfers	X				
Grades (current)	X		X		
Teacher evaluation					X
Trend indication	X		X		
Course load			X		
Learning line	X		X		
Delinquency/character disorders				X	
Sex-related problems	X		X	X	
Dropout/continuation of school	X			X	
Learning line (vocational future)			X	X	
Learning difficulty/ nonachiever	X	X		X	
Behavior change		X		X	

from stable and extreme, but also with which characteristics the differences were the greatest. The method offers two kinds of presentations of these hierarchically ranked variables discriminating among or between groups. One presentation is descriptive and empirical; it takes real distributions of student characteristics and change pattern groups and makes a "fit" showing how often one is able correctly to categorize students in these patterns by using all the variables that do discriminate. The second presentation uses these same variables to predict how well one can classify students into drug change groups when considering a new group of students about whom one has the same information. To accomplish both presentations using only one student population, it is necessary to divide that population into two matched subsamples.[a] The test of "fit" is made on the first half of the population, and the cross validation (cross verification or prediction test) is made on the second half. If both the fit and the predictions lead to assignment of students to categories (stable, common, and extreme) on a basis better than would occur by change expectancies, then one has assurance that the variables which are used in the equation are real discriminators.

The above are the elements of our procedure. The problems we encountered were of two kinds. One was the inadequacy of the file data, and the other was small sample sizes. With reference to the information in the student files, there are two sources of error. One is data omission. For example, while almost all files contained information on grades, most did not have information on learning difficulties, interest, leadership ratings, or the like. One cannot assume that the absence of an entry meant the absence of the trait, for it became evident that some teachers and schools kept more complete files than did others. A second error source is that of consistency and accuracy. Ratings of human beings by one another are notoriously unreliable. What is "leadership" to one teacher may be "aggressiveness" to another; undesirable behavior change seen by a teacher in one classroom may not show up in another. Our data showed us proofs of this unreliability even though we had no way in this study to describe its extent.

Because of reduced subsample sizes, we have limited analysis to the major use group, those showing sanctioned drug use at the time of first testing. To further increase sample size, levels 2 and 3 were combined so that these students are not differentiated by intensity of use. A further device employed, after examining the three patterns, stable, common, and extreme, was to contrast the two ends of the change distribution, stable versus extreme change, dropping out the middle (common) group. Only in cohort 10 was there sufficient initial variety of drug use to allow broader pattern comparisons. There we combined levels 4 and 5 into a beginning marijuana users sample whose stability and

---

[a]We took a list of all subjects, gave them sequential numbers, and made those with even numbers one half and the odd-numbered ones into the other half. Our total discriminant analysis sample was 1405, approximately half the size of our total research sample of 2908. This occurred because (1) we excluded all inconsistent students, and (2) we required that all students have a first and last test.

common, and extreme change were examined. We a so combined levels 6 through 9 into a high-risk group for a similar analysis.

Although there was but limited drug experience variability in the 2nd grade cohort (e.g., there were no children in the extreme change category), we did look for differences between stable and common change patterns. The 8th grade cohort was lost to us, for not only did we have only a small sample of students taught and tested over the full two years, but we were unable to collect complete clerical, file, and teacher data on the majority, because when they left the district to go on to 9th grade their file folders went with them to their new schools.

The 2nd Grade Cohort

Our attempt to classify 2nd grade cohort youngsters according to drug patterns, using data derived from routinely available administrative and teacher records, failed. The thirty-eight variables as reported by teachers and derived from the school files do not distinguish stable from changing drug use patterns among children in the 2nd grade cohort.

The 4th Grade Cohort

In the 4th grade cohort there were thirteen characteristics which formed a reduced variable set useful in discriminating one drug pattern from another.[b] Their nature and direction is as follows: *Major variables:* (1) More siblings in the family of extreme change students; (2) More positive attitudes toward school among stable students; (3) Few problems in peer relations among stable, more problems among extreme. *Minor variables:* (1) Common students were involved in more indoor activities; (2) Stable students participated more in interest activities; (3) The common group had more attendance problems;[c] (4) Extreme students were identified as suspected drug users;[d] (5) Stable students had changed schools more often; (6) Extreme students had had more favorable academic performance reports; (7) Extreme students had more sex problems; (8) Common students had more character defects and delinquency; (9) Extreme

[b]The cutting point was a contribution to overall variance of less than .01. Only three variables were consistently most important in discriminating between the groups in the cross verification analyses.

[c]Attendance records, except for unusual cases, are not routinely available in the elementary schools' student files. Entries here are spontaneous observations of teachers.

[d]This item was unrelated to our testing program; any observation of suspected drug use was a spontaneous and independent teacher entry into the file. No teacher had any knowledge of our student drug report responses.

students are more often underachievers and unmotivated in school; and (10) Stable students had least behavior change over time, extreme students the most.

The picture which emerges is fairly consistent, suggesting that children whose drug use remains stable in grades 2-4 come from smaller families and are better adjusted in school and with their peers.

In addition to the items on the full and reduced variable lists, we added the child's experience in drug education itself, learning that in the 4th grade cohort educational experience does not discriminate. This means that drug education there has less influence on a child's being in one or another drug use pattern than do the other features listed.

The association of a characteristic with a pattern by no means guarantees that one can correctly classify all of the students in a cohort, for, as we have noted, file data were frequently not available.

Accuracy is increased considerably when one disregards the common pattern and either fits or predicts for the two ends of the continuum, stable versus extreme. For the "fit" on the odd half of the sample, one can correctly place 83 percent (17 percent error) of the students in the stable group and 64 percent in the extreme. For the even half, one does better overall, 74 percent accurately placed in the stable group and 93 percent in the extreme. Prediction using these same variables is generally less satisfactory; 79 percent of the odd half are correctly predicted for the stable pattern, but only 50 percent for the extreme. For the other half of the population, one predicts 87 percent of the stable group but only 14 percent in the extreme group. To create an overall accuracy measure—a method we use in the rest of this chapter for stable versus extreme—we average the four cases of the prediction. That yields an accuracy of fit of 75 percent, and, for prediction, of 57 percent. The latter is only slightly above chance expectancy.

The 6th Grade Cohort

The nature and direction of the set of discriminating items between stable, common, and extreme is as follows (note that several student characteristics have equal power as major predictors): *Major variables:* (1) Delinquency, character defects: least in stable, most in common, some in extreme; (2) Least family problems in extreme, most in stable; (3a) Most intact families in stable, least in extreme; (3b) Father's occupation: highest income-education in stable, least in extreme. *Minor variables:* (1) Attendance problems: least in stable, most in extreme; (2) Suspected drug use: none in stable, some in common, most in extreme; (3) Sex-related problems: more girls in extreme, fewest in common; (4) Report card history (trend): most downward grade trend in extreme, least in common; (5) Interests-crafts (arts-crafts, mechanics-cars): least in stable, more in common, most in extreme; (6) Interests (general participants): most in stable, least in extreme; (7) Leadership: least in common, most in extreme; (8) Behavior problems: least in stable, most in extreme; (9) Referral to agencies for problems: most referrals in common, least in extreme; (10) Excessive absences: most in stable, least in extreme; and (11) Current grades: highest average in stable, lowest in extreme.

The discriminators between stable and extreme are as follows: *Major variables:* (1) Early report card history (trend): most downward grade trend in extreme; (2a) Interests (general participant): least in extreme; (2b) Least intact families in extreme; (3) Excessive absences: most in stable, least in extreme. *Minor variables:* (1) Domicile status; most living with parents in stable; (2) More sex-related problems among girls in extreme; (3) Most interests-crafts (arts-crafts, mechanics-cars) in extreme; (4) Most indoor interests (math, reading, science) in extreme; (5) Most leadership in extreme; (6) Family, home relationship best in extreme; (7) Most behavior problems in extreme; (8) Most attendance problems in extreme; (9) Suspected drug use most in extreme; and (10) Referral to agencies for problems most in stable.

We see that characteristics which were associated with drug patterns in the 4th grade no longer discriminate in the 6th grade cohort. There are exceptions to the trend first seen in the 4th grade cohort that extreme drug change youngsters most often show problem behavior. What best discriminated when stable, common, and extreme groups were compared no longer always applied when only stable versus extreme were compared. The most telling inconsistency is the contrast between "attendance problems," found most often in the extremes on the three pattern comparisons, and "excessive absences," found most often in the stable group on the two-pattern comparison. Remarks in the student files (coded as attendance problems) yield the opposite results from the remarks of teachers during the end-of-study final interview. We cannot say whether the discrepancy stems from the different absentee habits of children in one versus another class, from differences in what teachers consider absenteeism to be, from teacher differences in willingness to volunteer or record such observations, or from the sparse and sporadic nature of absentee observations as these are spontaneously offered either on records or in the interview. The discrepancy here illustrates how flimsy data can be when one relies on school file information which is gathered by other than systematic, verified methods.

In spite of such difficulties, there are some trends. By counting "problem" indicators (i.e., those items rating adjustment and performance: character defects, home difficulties, etc.) and limiting ourselves to items discriminating stable from extreme, we find that, of the nine problem measures (in stable versus common versus extreme), the extreme group is in the expected, more troubled, direction in seven. When looking at the stable versus extreme comparisons, we see that of the ten measures, seven are in that same direction. This cumulative evidence points to more personal, school, and family problems in the extreme group.

What if we add to these traits the drug education experience of the children? We find here that educational experience is a powerful discriminator. Its inclusion on the list would put it at rank 3, equal to family-home relationship in discriminating power. In the two-group comparison (stable versus extreme) it would also be rank 3, equal there to excessive absences. The extreme group in both instances has lower mean values, indicating that being in the drug education control group is associated here, as in the Chapter 6 findings, with having an extreme drug change pattern.

Items may discriminate successfully, but our list of these items (the variable list) may still not account for sufficient variance to assure a fully accurate classification of children into drug use patterns. Accuracy in classifying students into patterns is good when only stable and extreme groups are compared, averaging 85 percent for four "fits" combined. It is less good for prediction, averaging about 74 percent. This gives assurance that the variables overall contain enough information to allow one to separate children according to their longitudinal drug use patterns in spite of the poor quality of teacher ratings.

The 10th Grade Cohort

The nature and direction of the set of discriminating items for the stable, common, and extreme groups is as follows: *Major variables:* (1) Attendance problems: least in stable, most in extreme; (2) Sex-related problems: most girls in stable, least in extreme; (3) Family-home relationship: least family problems in stable, most in extreme. *Minor variables:* (1) Current grades: highest grades in stable, lowest in extreme; (2) Referral to agencies for problems: most referrals in stable, least in extreme; (3) Father's occupation: highest education-income in common, lowest in extreme; (4) Family status: most intact families in stable, least in extreme; (5) Early report card history trend: most upward in stable, least in extreme; (6) Interests-crafts (arts-crafts, mechanics-cars): least interest in commmon, most in extreme; (6) Interests (general participant): least interest in common, most in extreme; (7) Most leadership in common, least in extreme; (8) Behavior problems: least in stable, most in common; (9) Excessive absences (truancy): least in common, most in extreme; (10) Delinquency-character defects: none in stable or common, most in extreme.

The discriminating student characteristics for stable versus extreme patterns are as follows: *Major variables:* (1) Attendance problems: less in stable, more in extreme; (2) Behavior problems: less in stable, more in extreme; (3a) Sex-related problems: more girls in stable, more boys in extreme; (3b) Family-home relationship: less problems in stable, more in extreme. *Minor variables:* (1) Family status: more intact families in stable, less in extreme; (2) Domicile status: more living with parents in stable, less in extreme; (3) Early report card history (trend): less downward trend in stable, more in extreme; (4) Interests-crafts (arts-crafts, mechanics-cars); more interest in stable, less in extreme; (5) Most indoor interests (math, reading, science): less interest in stable, more in extreme; (6) Interests (general participant): less participation in stable, more in extreme; (7) More leadership in stable, less in extreme; (8) Referral to agencies for problems: more referrals in stable, less in extreme; (9) Excessive absences: less in stable, more in extreme; and (10) Transfer history: more transfers in stable, less in extreme.

The findings are consistent. Personal, school, and family problems tend to be concentrated among the extreme drug users, with the common pattern, as before, midway between. Note that referral to service agencies is contrary to this trend.

One item, the rating of suspected drug use, is notable by its absence. It appears that high school teachers are not sensitive to changes in drug use which characterize the majority (i.e., the sanctioned users). This should not be surprising, for such use is ordinarily away from school or is clandestine. Nevertheless, other traits the teachers do observe and comment upon call attention to some of the same youngsters we independently identify as expanding their illicit drug use. As in the 6th grade cohort, the areas of teacher ratings and comments or school records which contain information allowing one to separate stable from unstable users are those of personality, family, school performance, personal interests, socioeconomic status, peer group roles, and sex-related conduct. The variety of features here linked to drug use patterns is consonant with findings from much prior research.

What about drug educational experience? When we introduce into the variable set a student's experience with drug education modes X, Y, or Z, we find that, when stable, common, and extremes are contrasted, drug educational experience is not even a minor discriminant. When we compare stable versus extreme only, education does emerge as a minor correlate of pattern membership. Those students in the control group, X, are more likely to remain stable in their drug use. This is the same finding as set forth in Chapter 6 for the 6th grade cohort and as a tendency across cohorts. It is corroborated here. The importance of the drug educational influence among 10th grade sanctioned drug users competes poorly with the other minor variables.

With regard to the percentage "fit" and error rate, including prediction using the two halves of the 10th grade cohort population for the sanctioned drug users, the accuracy of classification using the information contained in our variable list is, as with earlier cohorts, higher for the stable versus extreme than when all three patterns are examined together. There is an overall fit accuracy of about 73 percent and a prediction accuracy of 66.5 percent. Once again prediction of new populations (i.e., classification in advance) is less accurate than the description of known ones.

Only in the 10th grade cohort were sample sizes large enough for us to learn what variables discriminated among drug patterns for students whose beginning drug levels were higher than the sanctioned drug levels. We list the characteristics discriminating among the stable, common, and extreme groups for the marijuana users, as follows: *Major variables:* (1) Early report card history: least downward trend in stable, most in extreme; (2) Course load: more academic in stable, "softer" in extreme; (3a) Relationship with peers: most well liked in common, least in extreme; (3b) Most indoor interests (math, reading, science): least interest among stable, most among extreme. *Minor variables:* (1) School: more from school *S* in stable, more from school *W* in extreme; (2) Mother's occupation: higher socioeconomic level in stable, less in extreme; (3) Early report card history (grades): higher among stable, lower among extreme; (4) Interests-crafts (arts-crafts, mechanics-cars): most interest in stable, least in extreme; (5) Behavior problems: least in stable, most in extreme; (6) Attendance problems: least in stable, most in extreme; (7) Excessive absences (truancy): most in stable, least in extreme; (8) Current grade trend: most unchanged in stable, most upward in extreme; and (9) Course load: most academic in stable, "softest" in extreme.

The items discriminating between stable and extreme groups are as follows: *Major variables:* (1) Mother's occupation: higher socioeconomic level in stable, lower in extreme; (2) Current grade trend: more upward in stable, less in extreme; (3) Early report card history (trend): more upward in stable, less in extreme. *Minor variables:* (1) Interests-crafts (arts-crafts, mechanics-cars): most interest in stable, less in extreme; (2) Behavior problems: less in stable, more in extreme; (3) School: more stable in school *S*, more extreme in school *W*; (4) Early report card history (grades): higher grades in stable, lower in extreme; (5) Most indoor interests (math, reading, science): less interest in stable, more in extreme; (6) Relationship with peers: more adequate, well liked in stable, less in extreme; (7) Attendance problems: fewer in stable, more in extreme; (8) Excessive absences (truancy): more excessive in stable; and (9) Course load: more academic in stable, "softer" in extreme.

One sees that school performance factors (grades, attendance, courses) appear frequently to discriminate among the longitudinal patterns of beginning marijuana users. Early grade trends emerge among the most distinctive items. This suggests that a downward trend in grades over a student's lifetime academic career prior to the 10th grade will be associated with expansion of his drug use beyond marijuana by the high school years. The grade trend is, paradoxically, reversed in Grades 10 and 11, showing that a downward trend is by no means linked to unusual (and in this instance, high-risk) drug taking (any common or extreme patterns beyond level 4 and 5 must embrace levels 6 and higher). We interpret this in the light of the selection of "softer" subjects by the common and especially the extreme change groups, compared with the hard or "academic" (and by implication college preparatory) course election by those marijuana users who do not expand their drug use in high school. Those students moving into high-variety (and higher-risk) drug use are also opting out of academic competition, a trend which is detectable in their earlier grade history.

The definitions employed for "attendance problems" and "excessive absences" differed for high school as contrasted with elementary records. Our "attendance" rating in the high schools was derived from the district computer records. Our measure of excessive absences in the high school was an administrative report to the effect that a child was truant. This required that teachers note and communicate frequent absences to the school administration. Whether that was done or not depended on the teacher. One would expect that the "attendance problem" rating would include many more students than the more extreme "excessive absences" and that the latter would be only a subpopulation of the former. The discrepancy, again demonstrating the unreliability of school records, shows most attendance problems, as derived from district computer entries, in the extreme group, but most truancies in the stable group. We presume that the computerized daily attendance record is more accurate.

School performance related items stand out in discriminating those who move onward and upward from marijuana in high school. These students show more absences and less academic orientation. Other identifying features which discriminate these students are: leisure interests, residential neighborhood, the school, personality (conduct) problems, adequacy of social (peer) relations, and maternal occupational level. Along with the residence item, this maternal factor may reflect family income status.

With reference to the percentage "fit" and error rate for classification, accuracy is increased by excluding the middle ground of the common pattern. When this is done, the accuracy for fit, averaged for the four cases, is 90 percent. The accuracy for prediction is 70 percent.

Let us consider students in the three change patterns whose beginning levels of drug use were already very high—levels 6-9—when we first began testing. This group necessarily had less opportunity to expand upward, i.e., to spread as much over levels. In the 10th grade cohort, all of the extreme group are students who moved upward from levels 6 and 7. One would expect that these high-level drug users would be more difficult to separate by discriminant analyses. Among the other students examined, extreme, as compared with stable students, described movement to more varied and intense drug use. In this group, however, where beginning levels are all at 6 or above, some of the extreme group will be moving upward to levels where some of the stable members are already found. Thus, ending drug levels can be the same for both extreme and stable students. The only certain difference is drug change among the extreme group during our experimental period. Thus, it is not so likely that the variables on our list which have discriminated among lower-level patterns would continue to be serviceable.

The characteristics which do discriminate comprise a reduced variable set of fourteen items. The nature and direction of the set of discriminating items for the stable, common, and extreme groups is as follows: *Major variables:* (1) Attendance problems: least in common, most in extreme; (2a) Referral to agencies for problems: occurs in stable, not among common or extreme; (2b) Family status: least intact families in common, most in extreme; (3) Relationship with peers: least adequate and well liked in stable, most in extreme. *Minor variables:* (1) Father's occupation: lowest socioeconomic level in stable, highest in common; (2) Early report card history (trend): most upward in stable, most downward in common; (3) Interests-crafts (arts-crafts, mechanics-cars): least interest in stable, most in extreme; (4) Outdoor interests (sports-PE, animals-fauna): least interest in common, most in extreme; (5) Suspected drug use: some in stable, most in common, least in extreme; (6) Excessive absences (truancy): least in stable, most in extreme; (7) Course load: most academic in common, "softest" in extreme; (8) Delinquency-character defects: least among stable, most among extreme; (9) Learning difficulties-nonachiever: present in stable and common, least in extreme; and (10) Behavior change: worsening in common, less so in stable, least in extreme.

The items discriminating between stable and extreme groups are as follows: *Major variables:* (1) Interests-crafts (arts-crafts, mechanics-cars): less in stable, more in extreme; (2) Excessive absences (truancy): less in stable, more in extreme; (3) Attendance problems: less in stable, more in extreme. *Minor variables:* (1) Father's occupation: lower socioeconomic level in stable, higher in extreme; (2) Family status: less intact families in stable, more in extreme; (3) Early report card history (trend): more upward in stable, more downward in extreme; (4) Outdoor interests (sports-PE; animals-fauna): less interest in stable, more in extreme; (5) Relationship with peers: more adequate and well liked in extreme, less in stable; (6) Suspected drug use: present in stable, none in extreme; (7) Referral to agencies for problems: less in stable, more in extreme; (8) Course load: more academic in stable, "softer" in extreme; (9) Delinquency-character defects: less in stable, more in extreme; (10) Learning difficulties/non-achiever: some in stable, none in extreme; and (11) Behavior change: some worsening in stable, none in extreme.

Students in the extreme group have the poorest school performance but are otherwise no worse off, as defined in terms of conventional personal or family evaluations, than the stable students. With regard to the teachers' suspicions of drug use, keep in mind that all students considered here were in the high-risk drug use group, so that any identification as an illicit drug user is correct. In any event, the item does not discriminate, and, further, most students were not suspect in spite of their high levels of use.

What about the utility of these variables for classifying students into patterns? Using the reduced variable set (fifteen), the average accuracy for classifying stable versus extreme is 94 percent, while, for predicting, it drops to 65 percent.

Discriminating Beginning Levels of Use

We have tested the utility of characteristics in distinguishing among students categorized according to their patterns of drug use over time. We now inquire as to which of these same variables discriminate the static condition of levels of drug use at the time of first testing, that is, when students enter a cohort. Since our 10th grade cohort was the only one with breadth in the distribution of these beginning levels, we restrict our examination to that cohort. As before, we have combined levels 2 and 3, 4 and 5, and 6-9, so that we have those entering the cohort with sanctioned drug experience (alcohol, tobacco), with marijuana, and with the injectables, pills, and powders which we consider high-risk substances. To sharpen analysis, we have compared students entering the cohort as sanctioned drug users with those entering at levels 5, 7, and 9, the highest-intensity use levels for marijuana, amphetamines, barbiturates, hallucinogens, cocaine, and opiates. For this run, we used the full set of thirty-eight variables, ordering all items by their power to discriminate among the subset of the ten most powerful discriminants. The emerging characteristics are as follows for levels 2-3 versus 4-5 versus 6-9: *Major variables:* (1) Behavior problems: least problems in sanctioned, most in high risk; (2) Course load: most academic in sanctioned, "softest" in high risk; (3) Feelings about school: most negative in sanctioned, least negative in high risk. *Minor variables:* (1) Early report card history (grades): highest grades in sanctioned; (2) Family status: least intact families in sanctioned, most in high risk; (3) Outdoor interests (sports-PE, animals-fauna): least in sanctioned, most in marijuana; (4) Suspected drug use: none in sanctioned or marijuana, some in high risk; (5) Interests-crafts (arts-crafts, mechanics-cars): most interest in sanctioned, least in marijuana; (6) Relationship with peers: most problems in marijuana, least in high risk; and (7) Learning line: English as a second language in marijuana, not in others.

The emerging characteristics are as follows for levels 2-3 versus levels 5, 7, and 9: *Major variables:* (1) Early report card history (grades): higher grades in sanctioned; (2) Behavior problems: more in higher-level use; (3) Leadership: greater leadership in sanctioned; (4) Learning line: most English as a second language in high-level use; (5) Ethnic background: more Caucasians in higher levels; and (6) Attendance problems: more among high-level users.

In this analysis the new items now operating are ethnic. More whites are found in the high drug use levels but so, too, are more non-English speakers (Spanish speaking). Perhaps these Hispanic students are present sufficiently in the white group to account for this ethnic-linguistic association with high-risk use. There is no consistent correspondence between negative personal or social evaluations and high-risk drug use, for while conduct problems are more common among high-risk users, peer relationships are described as poorest among the low-level sanctioned users. What is consistent is academic performance; low-level drug users have higher grades in their prior histories and show fewer current attendance problems. Suspected drug use is also associated with actual prevalence and incidence of use. Insofar as teachers in these high schools do suspect illicit use, those they suspect will be among the high-intensity and -variety users.

When the accuracy rate is calculated for degree of fit, one finds that for levels 2-3 versus 4-5 versus 6-9 it is 74 percent, and for levels 2-3 versus 5, 7, and 9 it is 56 percent. No predictive mode was employed.

The discriminant analysis shows that different features operate to distinguish among levels of drug use upon entrance into the 10th grade cohort as compared with patterns of change over time. Furthermore, the set of characteristics useful in distinguishing between levels not separated for intensity of drug use are partly different than the set needed to discriminate intensity levels. These observations indicate that within the 10th grade cohort there is considerable heterogeneity; each time one classifies drug use according to new criteria it is likely that new variables will appear which describe the students in those new classifications. The nuances of drug use classification are by no means inconsequential for the distribution of individual traits within patterns. Within general groups created for the purposes of analysis or discussion are found distinct subpopulations.

Resumé

Insofar as our goal has been to predict drug change on the basis of information ordinarily available in school files, or through brief interviews with teachers and school administrators, this has been modestly achieved. It is achieved most readily if one classifies students according to those who will be stable as opposed to those who will show the greatest increase in intensity or variety of drug use. Classification accuracy depends upon the age of the children and the drug use level at which one finds them. We show this graphically in Figure 7-1.

Reviewing the characteristics that have discriminated stable from changing students, we find that the major variables which discriminate patterns at one grade level need not apply to another grade level. For those entering a cohort as sanctioned drug users, for example, there is no characteristic which is of major importance for all four cohorts. Limiting ourselves to the three cohorts 4, 6, and 10, where our discriminating capability is most soundly based, three general themes are identifiable: school performance and adjustment, personal adjustment and interests, and some attributes of the family.

Within a cohort, patterns of change are differentially discriminated depending upon the entering drug use levels of students. For the 10th grade cohort, with its analysis for three entering levels, no major variable is common. Yet once again there are shared themes: school performance and adjustment, personal adjustment, and family attributes. Their item content is too diverse to justify a generalization, beyond noting that observations by teachers in the student file or observations that are clerically entered there which touch upon family attributes, school performance-adjustment, and personality or individual adjustment, all do reflect about the child something which is linked consequentially to his drug use over time.

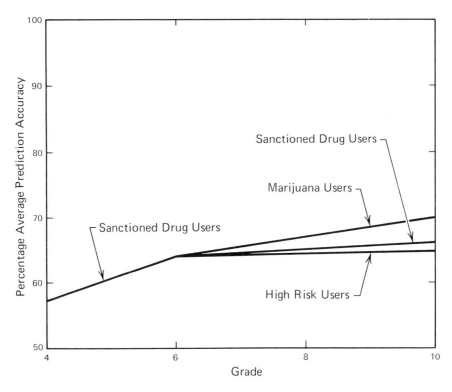

Figure 7-1. Accuracy of Prediction of Stable or Extreme Drug Use Patterns

Attending to all discriminating variables in the limited sets, there is one item that serves to discriminate across cohorts 6 and 10: excessive absences. Characteristics discriminating across cohorts 4, 6, and 10 for sanctioned drug users include character defect-delinquency, leadership, suspected drug use, interest in indoor activities, and interest in general participation. Only one of these is consistent in the direction of association: children rated by teachers as having character defects and/or as being delinquents are found among the increasing drug use group.

There are other items which remain consistent, or develop in logical fashion, even though they may not appear as discriminants at each cohort level. The current and early (all prior years) grade average is higher for the stables and worse for the extremes whenever it appears as a discriminator. Students in the extreme group take the nonacademic or "soft" courses in contrast to students in other patterns, and are also identified as those least often referred to service agencies. Only one feature consistently characterizes the common change group, whenever it appears as a discriminant, and that is having fathers in the highest socioeconomic level.

The foregoing trends favor an association between the expansion of drug use intensity and variety and a lifetime history of poorer grades, more evident behavior problems, and less academic competititveness for future higher education and professional careers. The presence of such trends does not efface great variability among individuals. Even being in the very highest levels by no means guarantees that an individual will be rated negatively by his teachers on matters of conduct, social relations, and personality. Neither rapidly expanding drug use nor a high level of use is inevitably correlated with adverse information. One of the consistent variables underscores that extreme students are at least often referred to service agencies or professionals for reasons which appear in the file to be negative, i.e., the presence of intellectual, personal, or familial difficulties. Were high drug levels and "troubles" to be equated in an easy stereotype, the reverse should have been true. Case review shows the majority of these referrals to have been for reading, speech, and health problems. Had the schools more habitually made referrals for emotionally disturbed or delinquent behavior, perhaps this finding would have been altered.

With regard to drug education, when that experience, whether in an X, Y, or Z class, is incorporated into the discriminant analytic procedure, the 6th is the only cohort for which that educational mode plays a role as a major characteristic equal to school, personal adjustment, and family features. One implication is of successful competition on the part of the school with these other drug conduct influences at about ages eleven through thirteen.

Remarkable Absences? A Query for Teachers

There are two potential actions by teachers with reference to drug-using students which are curiously absent. One is the identification of extreme drug users as such, and the other is their referral to helping agencies. We do not argue a need for the latter on grounds of drug use per se, but because the constellation of features associated with that use indicates that proportionally more of these extreme students do stand out as having greater problems in school and in personal-social adjustment. Absenteeism, downward grades, and undesirable conduct are noticed by the teachers even though teachers are not aware of the actual correlation of these with extreme drug patterns. That notice can begin as early as the 4th grade.

In any event, why is there not some better record on the part of school personnel in noticing troubles and making referrals to school counselors, mental health agencies, police juvenile bureaus, and the like? It cannot be argued that teachers are insensitive; even on the basis of the weak school records and unsystematic ratings that comprise our data base, they do prove sensitive. But they do not seem to have a means by which their sensitivity can be channeled into referrals.

What about other variables which were examined but did not discriminate? Consider the full set of thirty-eight. No more than fourteen account for most of the variance on any one run; the rest drop by the wayside. All in all, thirty-three appear as discriminants at some point in the analysis. Are there any that surprise us by their absence? Ethnicity could be one, for color and surname contribute in only one analysis to fitting or predicting the drug use change patterns. Health status ratings do not contribute either. Yet, if drugs are as dangerous as the folklore of anxiety and outrage holds, would not high intensity users be visibly ill, wasted, or otherwise suffering? They seem not to be, at least as far as teachers can perceive. The question here is whether or not extreme drug use does yield symptoms in the classroom which school authorities fail to see. Is teacher education deficient in alerting school personnel to drug phenomena? Or is it that most drug use is irrelevant as far as class conduct is concerned and that attention should be focused on those other correlates of school and personal performance?

The Influence of Family Characteristics

We conducted a substudy of the relationship between family characteristics and children's drug use. This was a test of the conclusions reached in our earlier work, *Horatio Alger's Children* (Blum and Associates, 1972a), to the effect that family factors do play a role in children's drug use patterns. We wanted to see if earlier findings from high school and college students' families, as derived from one set of methods, would be confirmed when different methods of observation were used with families of elementary school children.

The present study used a shortened inquiry form of 218 items, mostly direct questions to the mother, but also included were a few value- and goal-ranking tasks (for both mother and father[e]) and a few ratings of the home and activities there. Because in the earlier study we had spent many hours with all family members, we expected some differences in results, for Niemi's (1974) work has shown that perceptions by different family members can be quite adverse. There is, for example, only about 40 percent agreement between a wife's statement of her husband's stance on labor unions and the husband's own opinion elicited directly from him. A special problem in examining the association of our family items with drug use levels arises because there is relatively little variability in drug use levels and patterns among elementary school children as contrasted with the greater complexity of drug conduct in our earlier teenage sample. Only twenty-eight children, or 12 percent of those whose families were interviewed, reported drug use at level 4 or above as they entered the cohort (i.e., the time of our first testing). This drug use homogeneity made it impossible to array a distribution of children with very high versus very low drug use levels and at the same time to obtain the large sample sizes needed in testing for significant differences.

---

[e]Only twenty-four of the fifty-one fathers completed the forms.

Screening the Variables

We elected to compare the most extreme groups, although this inevitably led to only small samples being available for statistical tests. To screen the 218 items on a one-at-a-time basis, we used the "t test" to compare the average scores of the two groups. The two groups compared were the twenty-eight children with entering drug use levels of 4 and above (any marijuana use up through heroin-cocaine) and the twenty-eight youngsters who entered their cohort as abstainers. The 184 children at entering levels 2 and 3 were excluded from this analysis.

Abstainers Versus High-Level Users

Sixteen items (plus age-grade level) proved to be associated with high versus low levels of use at the 0.05 probability level; another seven emerged with probabilities in the 0.05 to 0.10 range. Thus, there are twenty-four family features which distinguish between children entering their cohort as abstainers versus those entering as users of the unsanctioned drugs, i.e., marijuana, stimulants, etc.

Drug-abstaining children more often, and high-level drug users less often, come from families where all the children are from the present marriage (i.e., are more often with their biological parents, less often with divorced or stepparents, etc.). Abstaining children more often have church-attending mothers and mothers who use little or no alcohol. Their mothers' leisure time activities less often incline to photography as a hobby and to collecting. There are more nonsmokers in the families of abstaining children, fewer fathers who use or have used barbiturates (prescribed or otherwise), and more mothers who have renounced or given up any further use of sedatives. The households of abstaining children's parents are more likely to require the children to perform household duties or chores, and parents in these homes have been away from their children while children were young for shorter periods of time than occurs in the homes of high-level users. The abstaining child is less likely to be rated by his mother as interested in trying new things or in sports participation than is the high-level using child. Parents of abstaining children are more likely to be in agreement on how and when to discipline their children than are parents of high-level using children, and these abstainers' parents also place a higher value on disciplining the child as contrasted with the high value placed by the other parents on children having independence and free choice. Freedom of choice is in fact given at an older age in the households of the abstaining children, at least when the measure is the age at which girls are allowed to choose whether or not they will join the family on vacations.

The values that parents wish to develop in their children differ. Families of abstaining children more often emphasize that children should love their parents and do not consider it valuable that the child be free to do what he wants. More often there is opposition in the abstainer's home to a child's trying marijuana than in the homes of the high-level users. Abstainers' mothers are more traditional in ranking child rearing goals, that is, do not emphasize the importance of preparing the child for a world of change. When asked what advice they would give to new parents, the abstainers' mothers are much more likely than other mothers to stress the need for direct physical supervision of a child by parents.

On two household rating items, the abstainer homes were ones labeled as neater and tidier than the others, and, during the interview for this study, the television was more often on there than in high-level user homes. There is one variable only among the twenty-four in which the direction of the findings here differ from that observed in our original study; it is the value placed by the father on teaching the children regard for law and order. In our earlier study, low-risk parents wished to inculcate a respect for the law, had good traffic obedience records, and had tolerance for police careers for their children. These were all features positively correlated with low-risk drug use in their children. Here we find the law and order variable reversed. The fathers of high-level users in this sample more often rank it important for children to learn respect for law and order than do abstainers' fathers.

Only a few of those family characteristics shown in our early study to be correlated with family features maintain a statistically significant association with children's drug use levels when tested under the conditions of the present research. The ones that do maintain predictive power under the less stringent probability level of $P < 0.10$ suggest that elementary school children whose drug levels are high, as compared with those whose levels are low, come from homes where parents seem less conventional, less religious, and more permissive, and thereby not only allow their children more freedom but believe that their children should be free and flexible. These families have children who seem to be more curious and adventuresome, and put less stress on child self-discipline and self-control. Parents of the high-level drug-using children supervise their children less and spend less time with them (and presumably, thereby, exert less control over the choice of peers and peer activities), use more psychoactive drugs themselves (socially, medically, and, as other studies have shown, illicitly), and are less opposed to illicit drug use experimentation by their children. These high-level users are under less obligation to love their parents and are living in families where the biological parents themselves may have loved one another less, as inferred from the greater prevalence of divorces, separations, and stepparents in these homes.

For every item shown here to be associated with high or low drug use levels, there were several others of a related nature, ones theoretically expected to reflect the same general theme, which did not prove significant. Clearly, it will take more study of families before one can identify the range of constellations which link drug use to family influences. Nevertheless, insofar as there are distinctive influences in the home, one sees how more varied, intensive, and illicit drug use can come to characterize some children and not others. Certainly those children who are encouraged by a home environment to be curious, unconventional, and undisciplined, who have more time for unsupervised peer activities, and who have parents who are themselves drug-using models not opposed to their children's illicit drug use, should find illicit drug experimentation perfectly compatible with what they have learned at home. These children may also be more unsettled psychologically insofar as greater family instability, lack of direction, and parental disagreement over the central features of child rearing do affect a child's mental health. Certainly we have no direct evidence of this from these interviews, although we do have evidence of the greater prevalence of problem children in the extreme drug change groups. The data support the possibility that there are at least two kinds of children entering the high-level and extreme change groups. One group would be those stressed and/or inadequate youngsters who have personal, social, and school problems and whose drug use may well be symptomatic of difficulty. The others would be children whose drug use is a possibly incidental outcome of their developing in those exploratory directions approved and sought by their parents.

Discriminant Analysis

Our next step in data analysis was to take the twenty-four family variables, plus the age-grade level variable, and to run a multiple discriminant analysis. This was done to screen and rate correlated variables and to devise a predictive equation. For the first round, we examined the success of classification, using these twenty-four variables to fit the fifty-one students into either the abstainer (level 1) or unsanctioned (levels 4 and above) groups. To test for both fit and prediction we divided each group (the low and the high levels) into two by assigning every other member of each into a subgroup; this was the same splitting procedure described earlier. In order to estimate the importance of the variable, we have summed and averaged the rank of each according to its power to aid in classifying in the (1) fitting, and (2) cross verification predicting modes. The seven most powerful variables, excluding grade in school and their relative ranks, are as follows:

Rank 1: Mother's rating of child's interest in trying new things
Rank 2: Value father places on child's learning high regard for law and order
Rank 3: Mother's opposition to child's trying marijuana
Rank 4: Absence of parental disagreement over child discipline
Rank 5: Age for girls with regard to freedom of choice whether or not to join the family on vacation

Rank 6: Interest of mother in collections as hobby
Rank 7: Requirement that child do work around the house

The most powerful family variable, averaged across fit and predictive modes, is the mother's rating of the child's interest in trying new things, a rating we equate with curiosity or adventuresomeness.

The accuracy of the fit of children in the abstainer or high-level use group, using this set of twenty-four variables, is excellent. All abstainers were correctly classified, all but one high-level user were correctly classified (one high-level user was incorrectly placed in the abstainer group). The overall error rate for fit is 0.02 percent, or 98 percent accuracy. In the predictive mode the average accuracy is 78 percent.

The accuracy of fit here is greater than that achieved in early tests of fit in Chapter 7. The quality of our data here on family features is much better than spontaneous teacher reports and unreliable school records. On the other hand, our sizes here are much diminished and drug use is less varied than in the full school populations analyzed earlier in this chapter.

Stable Versus Extreme Students

As another test of family features, we compared two other subgroups from our sample. One group ($N = 70$) consisted of families of students who entered the cohort at levels 1-2 (abstainers and sanctioned drug users) and remained at these levels. The other group ($N = 33$) consisted of families whose children entered at these same levels but who increased their variety or intensity of use over time to level 4 or higher. Level 4 was set as a cutoff point because we did not have enough students showing extreme changes—the most unusual 10 percent—to constitute an adequate sample.

There were nineteen items which discriminated the two groups at probability levels of 0.10 or lower, of which thirteen were significant at $P = 0.05$ or less.

When we compare these family traits with the characteristics shown earlier to discriminate children entering each cohort as abstainers versus high-level users, none are the same. The complete absence of overlap demonstrates that the subgroups of abstainers versus high-level users are quite distinct from the stable versus extreme group as to their separability on the full set of family variables.

The accuracy of classification for fit is, on the average, 78 percent, and for prediction, also 78 percent. Classification for fit remains higher than accuracy rates using teacher rating and school records. It is likely that there are family background differences among children when they are classified according to their variations in patterns of drug use, even when these variations appear minor.

The nature and direction of items which discriminate between stable and extreme children's families are as follows: Most powerful, in rank (1) is the mother's rating of the child's overall interest in illicit drugs; the extreme children are more interested; (2) Extreme parents are more in agreement on how the child's room should be kept; (3) More disagreement among extreme parents on the child's freedom to smoke; (4) Extreme parents allow freedom at an earlier age for boys to choose their own friends without parental supervision; (5) Extreme fathers use fewer sleeping pills; and (6) Extreme fathers place less emphasis on their children learning to get along with others. Less important discriminators are as follows: (1) There is more alcohol use by extreme fathers; (2) Extreme fathers have jobs in lower socioeconomic levels; (3) Extreme mothers use more tranquilizers and antidepressants; (4) Extreme mothers had more problems during childbirth, more worries about the child during infancy, and the child had greater health problems during infancy; (5) There is more disagreement between extreme parents over the child's use of leisure time; (6) There is more disagreement between extreme parents over the child's freedom to choose his own friends; (7) There is less emphasis among extremes by the father on the importance of the child learning to treat people as equals; (8) There is more frequent rating by extreme mothers that the child has used illicit drugs; (9) Segregationists are more emphasized by extreme mothers as posing problems to the nation; (10) Extreme mothers less often than stable rank Big Business as a group posing problems to the nation.

Interpreting this odd-lot group of findings, we infer that parental disagreement, parental drug use, infant health, the father's values, and the age at which freedom is granted to the child for choosing his own friends are all family background features linked to drug use stability. The mother's perceptions of her child's readiness to use and experience unsanctioned drugs is a powerful discriminator. Since it describes what we already know about the youngsters, this is not new information, but it does indicate that the mothers' estimates of their offsprings' relative drug use propensities may be accurate.

The direction which the discriminating items take usually parallels but occasionally diverges from that seen in *Horatio Alger's Children.*

For Educators to Consider

The reaffirmation that family background is linked to children's drug use in specific and predictable ways is something for school personnel to keep in mind. Since what parents do, value, and strive for may well be influential for their offsprings' drug conduct, should not parents themselves be taught what it is they can do which can affect their children's conduct? Isn't there a job for the school in teaching "parenting" and in giving child guidance information to those parents who want it? Would it not be a sound practice to invite parents to workshops, lectures, or even drug education planning seminars where parental influence and school activities might be joined?

If the family is as important as we think it is, might it also not be well for educators to hold out only modest hopes for the school's intervention? If, further, the family is but one of several powerful forces outside the school ground—personality, peers, neighborhood, income, culture—which affect drug conduct, is it not well for drug education personnel to be well acquainted with the scientific literature detailing the relationship of these forces to child behavior? Be that so, then adequate teacher education should be a necessary precommitment to any drug education for youngsters.

Summary

We employed a discriminant analysis technique to determine if student characteristics derived from school files and teacher commentaries distinguished among various drug change patterns over time. They did not do so for the 2nd grade cohort, but did so for the 4th, 6th, and 10th grade cohorts. There were not sufficient file data available on the 8th grade cohort to include them in the analysis. Sample size difficulties restricted us to those youngsters entering each cohort as sanctioned drug users, except in the 10th grade cohort, where those entering as marijuana users and as high-risk users (levels 6 and above) were included.

In the 4th grade cohort, those sanctioned drug users whose drug use remained stable were better adjusted in school and with their peers. In the 6th and 10th grade cohorts, those that showed the most extreme drug changes had more personal, school, and family problems. Among the 10th grade marijuana users, school performance loomed largest as a discriminating item, with the more extreme users not only showing present difficulties, but also having report card histories in their earlier years that more often showed a downward trend. Personal and social problems were also more often present among those showing the most extreme increases in use. Discrimination among the already high level users in the 10th grade cohort was not consistent except for poorer school performance among the extreme change group. Drug education experience as a variable appeared powerful only at the 6th grade cohort, corroborating Chapter 6 findings that membership in the control, X, educational group was associated with extreme drug shifts (spread). With reference to the quality of the discriminant analysis technique, the best predictions were obtained for all cohorts when stable students were contrasted with extreme change patterns, with the more common changes excluded.

Examining specific characteristics, there was no major variable which discriminated patterns across all cohorts (excluding cohort 2) and entering levels within cohorts. The major themes, however, of personal adjustment, personal interests, and family attributes did appear. Among all discriminating variables, only one appeared across all cohorts and levels, that being excessive absences.

This item has, however, been shown to be unreliable when teachers' records are compared. Only one item showed a consistent direction across all cohorts: the teacher rating of character defects-delinquency was always associated with increasing drug use, in contrast to stable use. Across all the entering levels of the 10th grade cohort, items consistent in their direction were early report card trends, attendance problems and excessive absences, and conduct (behavior) problems. These were associated with increasing as opposed to stable drug use patterns. Characteristics which were consistently more often present among extreme change groups were lower early grade averages and a greater proportion of "soft" as opposed to "academic" courses. This group also showed the least referrals to service agencies. In the classification of drug change patterns neither ethnicity nor teachers' ratings of health distinguished among students.

When the discriminant analysis method was applied to entering drug use levels in the 10th grade cohort, a static measure not linked to change patterns, differing characteristics were found to serve as discriminants depending on both kind of drugs and intensity of use. More whites and native Spanish speakers are in the high-use levels, while low-level users have the better academic performance. Teachers correctly suspect illicit drug use among those in fact engaged in greater illicit use.

Our basic data for the foregoing analyses are weak because student file data are inconsistently entered and the reliability of teacher ratings is suspect. With these limitations in mind, we can nevertheless conclude that the student characteristics routinely observable by teachers do distinguish student characteristics which are correlates of drug use change patterns and entering drug use levels. The general direction of ratings finds the more rapidly expanding drug users to have more problems in school, with their peers, and in society. However, there is no simple relationship between the presence of such difficulties and either the static level of drug use or the risk of rapidly increasing use. No safe inferences as to cause and effect can be derived from our data.

In a substudy of family factors, interviews were conducted with the mothers of 235 children drawn randomly from the 4th, 6th, and 8th grade cohorts. A brief questionnaire was filled in by only about half of the fathers. Inquiry items were derived from our earlier (Blum and Associates, 1972a) study of family factors distinguishing between high, medium, and low drug risk youngsters. Twenty-three children entering their cohort as abstainers were compared with twenty-eight whose entering levels were 4 and above (unsanctioned substances). Sixteen items discriminated at the 0.05 probability level, another seven in the 0.05-0.10 range. The number of significant variables emerging from this study is not impressive, since some will achieve significance by chance alone.

Our inference from the items was that the parents of the abstainers, compared with parents of high drug level children, were more religious, enjoyed greater marital stability and agreement, used fewer drugs, placed greater emphasis on child rearing, work, duty, discipline, and love of parents, supervised their children more closely, were more conventional, and opposed unsanctioned drug use. The higher drug use level children were, on the other hand, more often characterized as curious and adventuresome and their parents appear to value freedom, flexibility, and independence in the child. The multiple discriminant analysis procedure used here yielded higher rates of accuracy for fit and prediction than were obtained in the classification (fit and prediction) of children's drug use based on teacher ratings and school records. This can most likely be accounted for in part because of the better quality of data from this substudy.

A second analysis of family features compared seventy stable with thirty-three extreme drug-using children, again from the family substudy total of 235 mothers and fathers. Except for school grade, the variables which discriminated these two groups were different than those distinguishing abstainers from high-level users. This suggests that subgroups of children that are defined differently by rather refined measures of drug use are in fact different in family background. Said another way, the population of drug-using children is hetero-geneous, and, in consequence, subgroups created by different criteria for drug use classification may reflect separate sets of influences and have different family correlates.

The discriminating items suggest that the families of extreme drug-using children show more alcohol and tranquilizer use (but not more sleeping aids), that parents disagree more on child rearing practices bearing on the child's leisure time, drug use, and choice of friends, that an early "trouble" variable in infancy may exist, and that a sociopolitical stance which is antidemocratic may be present. The highest-ranked discriminator is the mother's rating of her child's overall interest in unsanctioned drugs. This, coupled with another discriminating rating, the mother's estimate of the child's actual drug use, indicates that mothers' judgments of their children's drug propensities are likely to be correct.

For the most part, these themes, as we infer them from the discriminating items, are similar to the results of our early, more detailed and intensive family study reported in *Horatio Alger's Children*. A discrepancy does exist here in the association of possible antidemocratic social views with greater children's drug use, as contrasted with the relationship between political conservatism and reduced drug risk in the earlier study. If, however, political conservatism of agreeable families and social traditionalism are distinct from a reactionary spirit in interpersonally disharmonious families this discrepancy becomes explicable. We must not, in any event, expect too simple a formulation to link family influences to different levels and patterns of children's drug use. Not only are results likely to differ as methods and samples change, but the diversity of drug use patterns, shown now to be associated with differing child characteristics either in terms of family features or teacher ratings and school records, warns us that complexity and diversity must be assumed when one seeks to classify and comprehend the etiology of children's drug use. We do, nevertheless, propose that a variety of family features are influential on that drug use. Be that so, then educational intervention is aimed at behavior which has been set in motion by forces at work earlier in life than school attendance and most likely operating outside the school, i.e., in the home itself. Drug educators should keep the importance of parents in mind.

8

Inhalant Users: A Special Case

Inhalant Use

This chapter presents information on the use of inhalants[a] in our sample, and its relationship to drug education and to student characteristics. Our consideration of inhalants is separate from other psychoactive substances because their use and correlates are somewhat different; there is not a continuously rising prevalence and incidence in use in our population throughout grades and ages. Furthermore, using our classification scheme, there is less order or scalability such that the use of one drug at a particular level implies the likelihood of the use of all other lower-level drugs.

The Prevalence of Inhalant Use

Figure 8-1 shows the proportion of students in each cohort who, by their final test, report experience with inhalants. More students in the 6th grade cohort than any other have had experience with inhalants; the trend is not one of rising use for older youngsters. To the contrary, less than half as many high school students report having had any lifetime experience with these substances as do those in grades 6-8. This, in turn, suggests an historical or fashion-dependent as well as age-linked occurrence.

Problems in Report Accuracy

The foregoing findings can be in error if the reports on the lifetime history of use upon which we relied have underreported past use. We examined the responses of youngsters on the self-report and did find evidence of error greater than that seen for reports of other drugs. One error measure is the comparative

---

[a]Inhalants, or volatile intoxicants, were defined for our purposes as any of those materials which are sniffed to achieve real or imagined central nervous system effects inferred to be desirable experiences by the users. The definition excludes anesthetics medically administered, but would include anesthetics obtained and used outside of medical supervision. It excludes substances enjoyed only for their odors. Typically included are airplane glue, gasoline, nitrous oxide, aerosol hair sprays, antiasthmatics (not being used to treat congestion), paint thinner, etc. With the exception of anesthetics, inhalants are usually manufactured products not intended for medical use and not ordinarily designated as "drugs."

125

126

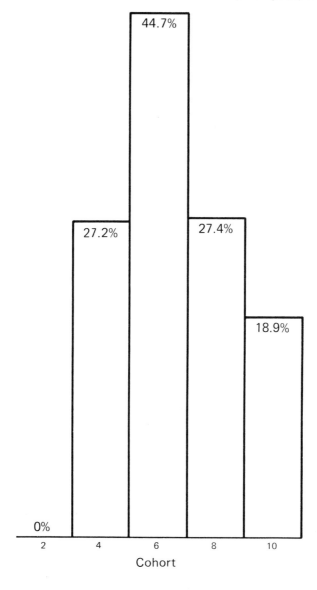

Percentage of Total Sample
Reporting Any Experience

Figure 8-1. Inhalant Use among Cohorts

reliability of the visual and written test forms. Our reliability analysis led us to conclude that the visual form is a poor test for eliciting inhalant use history as compared with the written form. The implication of the test unreliability is that there is more inhalant experience among the younger children than that reported in the visual test. This does not effect the data base of inhalant experience rates for the 5th and higher grades (cohorts 4, 6, 8, and 10) because the written test was used exclusively at grade 5 and higher. Another error estimate comes from looking at test inconsistencies. Examination of inhalant inconsistency rates shows that 39 percent of the 4th grade cohort, 42 percent of the 6th, 56 percent of the 8th, and 55 percent of the 10th were inconsistent.

We suspect that inhalant inconsistency rates are higher than rates for other drugs because the circumstances surrounding use can be ambiguous. With inhalants as with no other drugs, intention defines whether or not drug use has occurred. Children's reports are therefore in response to a more complex, two-part question. Consider the child using glue to build a model airplane. He necessarily smells the glue and may interpret what he has done as consonant with our question, "Have you ever tried sniffing things like glue or paint thinner with the intention of getting high?" Later, on another test, he may construe his actions to have been different, i.e., as inhaling without the intent to get a mental effect.

We can enter a precautionary correction which makes the worst assumption, that the inconsistency rates for each cohort reflects an error of measurement such that the "real" prevalence rate may vary above and below the highest reported rate to the extent of the error. The observed 18.9 percent rate for the 10th grade cohort, for example, would then range from approximately 9 percent to 29 percent since there is a 55 percent inconsistency rate for that cohort. Figure 8-2 offers alternative rates for inhalant use showing, by dotted lines, possible error. Figure 8-2 is derived from the special subsample of written tests and inconsistency data. Relative to one another, the prevalence rates for cohorts remain unchanged.

Inhalants in Combination With Other Drugs

We wanted to learn with what other drugs inhalants are combined during students' lifetime experiences. Examining the refined population of students taking the last test given in each cohort ($N = 1772$), we find that the majority of inhalant users (60 percent) in the 4th grade cohort had experience only with the sanctioned drugs (alcohol, tobacco). In the 6th grade cohort more inhalant users (41 percent) were in the group having used only sanctioned substances than were in any other group. In the 8th grade cohort, one-third of the inhalant users were

128

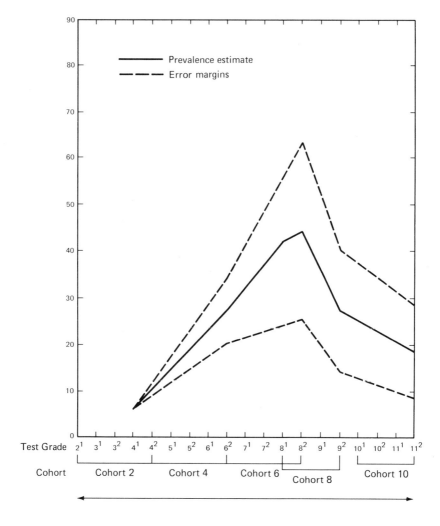

Figure 8-2. Estimated Prevalence of Inhalant Use by Grade, Utilizing Subsample Written Test and Margin Calculated on Inconsistency Rates

students whose only other use was of sanctioned drugs, and one-third were students who had used the sanctioned drugs plus marijuana plus amphetamines, and/or barbiturates and/or hallucinogens. In the 10th grade cohort, more (47 percent) of the inhalant users were found to have also used the sanctioned drugs plus marijuana and the amphetamine/barbiturate/hallucinogen cluster than any other combination.

Combining all cohorts, we find that of those reporting any inhalant use, 2 percent are otherwise abstainers reporting no self-administered use of any other psychoactive substance, and 45 percent report use of the sanctioned substances only. Twenty-nine percent report use of both sanctioned substances and marijuana, 3 percent use of sanctioned substances plus one or more in the amphetamine/barbiturate-hallucinogen class (but no marijuana), and 21 percent experience with all of the foregoing. This distribution is unlike the more predictable hierarchy of use characterizing the rest of our classification scheme. It does indicate that inhalant use nearly always occurs among students who have also used tobacco and/or alcohol, that half of the inhalant users will also have had experience with marijuana, and that one-fourth of them will have had experience with amphetamines/barbiturates/hallucinogens.

Inhalants and Longitudinal Patterns for Other Psychoactive Drugs

Using the entire population on which longitudinal pattern data are available, we examined the distribution of inhalant users. Inhalant users constitute 50 percent or more of the total found in all three of the extreme patterns which exist in the 4th grade cohort. For the 6th grade cohort the inhalant users constitute the majority of the four extreme patterns existing in that cohort. They also contribute all of the members to the only change pattern existing, common, among youngsters entering the cohort at level 6 (amphetamines, etc.). In the 8th grade cohort all of the youngsters in the extreme patterns emerging from the three highest beginning drug levels (5, 6, and 7), and two-thirds of those in the only pattern (stable) for beginning level 8, (heroin/cocaine) are inhalant sniffers.[b] In the 10th grade cohort, inhalant users contribute the majority to the two extreme patterns deriving from the highest beginning levels, levels 6 and 7, and to the two patterns which derive from those entering the cohort at the highest level for that cohort, level 8.

The foregoing shows that, without exception, inhalant-using students constitute the majority of children in all the extreme change patterns for the lower grades. They comprise all of those at the highest beginning drug levels who show any increase in their drug use during the years of the study. For the older students, grades 8 through 11, inhalant users comprise the majority both in the extreme patterns derived from the higher beginning levels and among those entering at the highest level for each cohort who show any increase in drug use. It is evident that younger students in any extreme change pattern, and older ones in the extreme patterns of those entering a cohort with already high levels of use, are both disproportionately drawn from among inhalant users.

---

[b]In this analysis using a larger population, there are inhalant users in the 8th and 10th cohorts reporting use of heroin-cocaine.

Only a small proportion from among all inhalant users contributes to the above-noted extreme and high beginning level common patterns. The proportions are: 19 percent in the 4th grade cohort, 15 percent in the 6th grade cohort, 18 percent in the 8th grade cohort, and 23 percent in the 10th grade cohort. Thus, while most of the rapidly expanding (extreme) users of other psychoactive drugs are inhalant users across all cohorts, less than one-fourth of all the inhalant users within any cohort are in the extreme and high beginning level patterns. This suggests that the inhalant users consist of at least two types of children, one type with the pattern of rapid drug use increase and the other enjoying more conventional drug use.

Educational Experience

We grouped inhalant users according to their drug educational experiences, modes X, Y, or Z. In the 4th grade cohort, there was no difference at the time of first testing; most reported no inhalant use at that time. The most common occasion for first use to be reported was at test 3 for the Y and Z group, whereas for the controls, X, onset is later, at test 5. About one-third of each group were inhalant users by the final test. The delay in onset among controls, while not significant statistically $(P > 0.05)$, suggests that minimal exposure to drug education may slightly delay, but nevertheless will not prevent inhalant experimentation in grades 4-6.

For the 6th grade cohort, there is inequality of experience among the education group at the time of the first test, presumably due to chance factors in assignments to classes. By the time of final testing, more X and Z students than Y have reported their first inhalant experience during the years of our teaching. This suggests an advantage in didactic, Y, education which may retard onset of inhalant experimentation. For the 8th grade cohort there is a slight tendency— not statistically significant[c]—for the Y group to delay onset of the first experience to a later time, as compared with the X and Z groups. The same delay in sniffing is observed (again not statistically significant[c]) in the 10th grade cohort. We conclude that there is no strong evidence for a preventive effect for one versus another mode of drug education, when prevention is defined as lower prevalence by the time of final testing. The trend, consistent through cohorts 6, 8, and 10, of a delay in the onset of inhalant experimentation in the didactic, group merits further investigation, as does the possibility of slower onset of experimental sniffing for students that receive minimal drug education in the early grades. Since there is very little high frequency inhalant use in our population—only 16 percent of all inhalant users—we can make no statements with reference to the possible role of drug education in retarding the spread (i.e.,

[c]Statistical testing here is limited by small sample sizes. A larger N might have yielded real differences.

rapid expansion) of inhalant use. The trends observed are fully consistent with findings in Chapter 6.

Characteristics Associated with Inhalant Use

We used the discriminant analysis method and the full thirty-eight-variable set to determine if inhalant users could thereby be distinguished from other students. Sufficient sample sizes were available only in the 4th and 6th grade cohorts. In both cohorts, stable and common low-sanctioned users were examined. No characteristics emerged as very powerful predictors, and, in the several analyses, the directions of association tended to reverse themselves. This indicates that the traits earlier found helpful in discriminating among psychoactive drug patterns are not very useful in separating out inhalant users as such. The only consistent discriminating variables suggest that inhalant users in grades 6-8 are more often nonwhite and have lower grades, but they are not identified by teachers as classroom, social, or personal "problem" youngsters. Given the absence of a consistent cluster of items, and the weak power and high variability yielded through this analysis, it is evident that teacher ratings and school records fail to show how inhalant users differ from other students.

Comment and Summary

Inhalant use stands apart from the social and private use of other psychoactive substances by the young people in our sample. Instead of steadily increasing prevalence by age and grade, experimentation with sniffing compounds (we say "experimentation" because most do not report frequent use) is at a peak in the 6th through the 8th grades. Furthermore, that peak seems to be a current fashion, for older students do not report as widespread a usage when they were in those same early grades. Reports of inhalant use appear to be more unreliable than those of other drugs.

Inhalant users contribute disproportionately to the group of students who rapidly increased their use of other drugs during our study. About one-fifth of all inhalant users account for this concentration in the extreme change patterns. This, in turn, suggests that there are at least two kinds of inhalant users; one is a special group whose inhalant use is linked to extensive and rapidly increasing other drug use, and the other is a group where, for the majority, drug experience is limited to conventional alcohol, tobacco, and marijuana. The combination of other drugs inhalant users are most likely to use is less easily predictable than is other drug use as pursued by our major classification scheme of levels and patterns. Even so, it is clear that these sniffers of volatile materials are users of other psychoactive drugs and, about half the time, are users of the illicit compounds in levels 4 and above.

Attempts to discriminate inhalant users from other students were for the most part a failure. Sixth grade cohort sniffers are more often nonwhite and have lower current grade averages, but they do not seem visible to teachers as being a school, social, or personal problem group. Had sufficient sample sizes been sufficient to separate out those inhalant users who were in the extreme patterns of drug use, better discrimination would have been obtained.

With reference to the impact of drug education, there is no strong evidence for the preventive role of any mode. Two trends are consistent with our other findings: (1) inhalant use in the 4th grade cohort with least drug education, and (2) the suggestion that didactic education may somewhat retard the onset of experimentation. It is not known what factors account for the rapid rise of inhalant use to peak in early years and then diminish in the older grades. Knowledge of these facilitating and restraining forces might help the general design of more effective drug education.

9 Consumer Evaluations

The consumers of our drug education endeavor were the students themselves and, as concerned parties, their parents. The teachers and administrators in the schools where we worked, along with the district administrators, were our friendly critics, for we undertook responsibility to do the teaching job which they were required to do by law. Insofar as our drug education curricula are said by us to be accurate, appropriate, and selectively effective, educators elsewhere considering the strategies we propose will want to know what the students and educators in the four California cities where we worked had to say. This chapter, therefore, reports the reactions of consumers to our product.

Students

During the last class session of our teaching, we distributed to all cohorts forms eliciting student reactions to our drug education programs. The questionnaire, in several versions geared to reading levels, was returned by 87 percent in the 2nd and 4th cohorts, 96 percent in the 6th, 75 percent in the 8th, and 66 percent in the 10th.

Class Enjoyment

Asked if they enjoyed their drug education classes, the majority in cohorts 2, 4, and 6 answered "Yes." The figures, averaged across the educational modes, were respectively 90 percent, 90 percent, and 82 percent. Reduction in consumer satisfaction begins to appear in cohort 8, where 60 percent stated they viewed the drug education classes positively, whereas in cohort 10 only 50 percent were satisfied with the classes. Observe that satisfaction peaked in the early cohorts where the greatest impact of drug education occurred. High school, where our statistics show no impact for drug education, is also where the students least liked the drug education classes.

There are no great differences between groups X, Y, and Z in any cohort. The greatest difference is 10 percent between Y and Z in the 10th grade cohort (46 percent versus 56 percent): the elementary school differences are on the order of 1-9 percent. This uniformity suggests that pupil sentiments about drug education are unrelated to the content, frequency, and style of our teaching.

Controls receiving factual information three times a year (this was the minimum allowable in conformity to state law) were just about as pleased or displeased as those in personally oriented discussion groups which met every two weeks. The same teachers did the teaching in each group, so we may be measuring a response to them. We know, given the great drop in high school satisfaction, that grade level is a big factor. That half of the high school students did enjoy classes and half did not also tells us that there are other factors influencing these reactions.

Enjoyment of Teacher

Evaluations of our teachers were overwhelmingly positive. The few negative responses (8 percent) were concentrated among high school students and in the one 8th grade class which contained students with a school-wide reputation for belligerence. The high school replies show that students can appreciate a teacher without enjoying the subject matter.

Did They Learn Anything?

The curve of acknowledged learning drops dramatically, from a high of 94 percent in grade 4 and 89 percent in grade 6, to 62 percent in grade 8, and to a low of 42 percent in grade 11. Only slight differences (maximally 16 percent, and ordinarily considerably less) separate the X, Y, and Z groups, although in the elementary school cohorts the control group consistently reports less learning. In high school, as many controls say they have learned something as do students in the Y and Z educational experience groups. Given grade differences in impact, these responses may be an accurate reflection of learning.

Asked what they had learned, most responding students referred to facts of a pharmacological nature. The pharmacological awareness figures were compatible with our education approaches, being greatest for the didactic modes and least for process modes. Consistent with the reported learning, from high in elementary school to low in high school, far more early grade children than high school students said they had acquired new scientific knowledge. We would expect self-perceived learning to depend on the type of educational experience, X, Y, or Z; for example, process students should sense they have learned something more about values and decision making than did cohorts. No elementary control school controls (X) and only 4 percent of the high school controls (spontaneously) mentioned learning in either of these areas. An average of 4 percent of the information (Y) classes in elementary school and none in the high schools indicated they had learned about values or decision making. In the Z classes, specifically oriented to decision making and value clarification, an average of 16 percent in elementary and 7 percent in the high schools said they had learned something about these areas.

Reported awareness of learning in response to drug education is strongly associated with grade levels. Perhaps by high school most students either insulate themselves from the drug educational process, maintain an attitude that they have nothing more to learn, or may in fact have nothing more to learn from us. Since our instruction in the control groups was minimal, we expected the controls to report comparatively less as having been learned. That they did not suggests that all of the elementary students felt that, by their own standards, they had learned something even if, according to our view, there were great differences between the amounts of knowledge the X, Y, and Z materials offered. It may also be that there is a readiness to learn and an attitude of acceptance among elementary school students which leads to a positive evaluation of any new material acquired; this attitude was not often found in the high school students. We did not expect the Z group to report pharmacological learning, for we did not intend to convey and the curriculum did not contain facts as such. Yet our elementary school Z students did—although to a lesser extent—feel they had learned pharmacological facts. Contrariwise, we expected the Z students to learn about values and decision making, but most did not mention these features.

That an average 12 percent more of Z than Y did say that they had learned about their values and decisions is reassuring, but not as important as finding out that what we thought we were teaching differed dramatically from what students described as what they were being taught. We cannot be sure whether this was due to a failure on our part to emphasize sufficiently the process components in Z, to a reluctance of students to acquiesce in the rather novel teaching approach of Z in favor of sensitivity to the remaining traditional components therein (implying educational conservatism in youngsters), or whether in their reporting youngsters simply chose to emphasize that they had learned facts about science rather than to express sensitivity to their own personal and peer processes; replies to the next question throw some light on this discrepancy.

Effect on Decisions

Students were asked if the drug education program had any effect on their own decisions about drugs. The great majority of younger students said "yes," while only a few of the high school students so stated. The decline in acknowledgement of the role of drug education in their personal decisions is quite regular with increasing age. Although there are variations from group to group, there are no consistent trends for children in any one educational experience to state that their decisions are more affected than those in other groups. One would have expected that the value clarifying, decision process-emphasizing Z group would yield youngsters who were much more sensitive to the decision process, providing that the development of drug use is subject to conscious decision making.

There is little research evidence to tell us what kind of conscious decision making occurs as children accept or reject drug-taking opportunities. Nor do we know how much awareness or recollection children have of cognitive events that might occur. Possibly, replies reflect the expectations of children as to what should occur. For example, if the younger children believe that such education is supposed to affect their decisions, they can say it does. If teenagers consider it unfashionable to admit of any decisive role for adult guidance in their pridefully autonomous (in fantasy, if not in fact) moral and social life, they will deny influence. Alternatively, replies may simply express the desire to acquiesce in what youngsters believe may be our, the testers', expectations. Conforming to and pleasing the authorities by agreeing that their efforts worked as intended can be age appropriate for a 4th grader but not for a rebellious high schooler. Nevertheless, the correspondence between the ages for actual drug education influence, as empirically validated, and children's assessments, suggests that something of what children tell us about influences on their decisions may be correct.

The Aim of Drug Education

Asked what their teachers had been trying to teach them, one finds that students in the process experience, more often than others, attributed to the teacher the intention of affecting the values and decision process. Five percent of those in the control group, 2 percent in the didactic group, and 14 percent in process education so characterized the teachers' aims. These figures are almost exactly the same as those for the open-ended earlier query as to what had been learned. We interpret them again in the same way: there is slight agreement between what we intended to do in *X, Y,* and *Z* and what the children thought we were doing. Most children did not tell us that they experienced the particular kind of drug education which we intended to provide. A constraint on our interpretation arises from the nature of the questionnaire itself, for it relied—on both these items dealing with *X, Y,* and *Z* content differences—on the spontaneous formulations of the children: they had to describe the experience as they saw it. Insofar as they were poor in generating such descriptions, and if it was more difficult for them to describe value, decision, and norm-setting intentions or learning, then the questionnaire method could be insensitive. Nevertheless, since the refinements that differentiate the kinds of drug education presented within our framework are not strongly mirrored in the descriptions, one must entertain the possibility that actual differential educational effects are not dependent upon a conscious awareness on the part of youngsters of the kind of educational method to which they are being exposed.

Suggestions for Improvement

About 10 percent of the students in each group suggested scheduling changes when asked what improvements were in order. Primarily these were requests for more frequent sessions. There were a greater number of such requests from the infrequent X group than from the more frequent Y and Z groups. With respect to course content, the least number of suggestions came from 2nd and 4th grade cohort members in the X group and high school students in the Z group.

Suggestions for outside speakers came most often from high school students, although not from any in the Z group. Some students at all levels and in all groups wanted more information on drug effects. Movies were most often proposed by younger students in the Y and Z groups. Discussion groups were proposed by a very few students, most of whom were older. Paradoxically, the greatest percentage of discussion group requests came from high school youngsters in the Z group. Our impression is that students did not easily generate new ideas for drug education. That the infrequently meeting controls were for the most part not desirous of more sessions suggests to us a rather passive acceptance of the whole business. That the high school students, in spite of their earlier statements that they had not enjoyed the courses and had not learned or been affected by them, were neither destructively critical nor constructively redesigning our work, makes us think that for all their expressed disdain for the content they were not as unhappy with it as might be thought and again were passively rather than actively involved. That some high school students in the Z group could propose that discussion groups were needed tells us once more that what we thought we were doing in school and what students saw us as doing can be miles apart. On the other hand, that more high school Z students (67 percent) wanted no changes and no outside speakers, as compared with the greater wish for change among other groups (X: 48 percent, Y: 55 percent), may mean that process education may not be as indistinguishable from other methods as their other comments would lead one to believe.

Should Drug Education Be Taught in School? Students answering "yes" to this question were asked what kind of program it should be. The greatest number saying both "yes" and then saying that the program should be the one they were experiencing were in the X group, 64 percent, followed by 56 percent of the Y and 50 percent of the Z. Much like replies to the earlier content suggestion question, most proposals for change called for more information on drug effects and for more movies. Only a few called for discussion groups, and, as with the earlier question, one finds that, paradoxically, as many students in the Z classes asked for innovation in the form of discussion groups as did other students. Asked what grade levels should receive drug education, grades 5-8 are most often selected, and grades 3-4 follow. High school is least recommended, along with kindergarten through grade 2. These student recommendations are that drug education be taught in those same grades, 5-8, where our empirical data has found it to be most effective; these are the same grades where students report that they have found it most enjoyable, have learned most, and have been most infuenced by it. There is an impressive affinity between our statistical data and the intuitive recommendations and experiential reports of students.

Who Should Teach Drug Education? Students liked our teachers. Answers to the question of who should teach were further proof. Almost all students—all cohorts and all groups—said they should be the same people or teachers similar to those who presented our Stanford drug education program.

Reasons For Changes in Drug Use. As part of testing we had asked students if their drug use had changed. When it had, we inquired about the reasons. How important did drug education loom, compared with other events in their lives? We asked those students indicating drug use change over the last several years to check, from a list of nineteen, the main reasons they felt led to this change. In order to eliminate bias arising from the high or low position of an item on the check list, we distributed three versions of this question, each with a different position order for the possible reasons for change. The check list responses ($N = 1332$) reveal the first-ranked response—the change most often cited—as "having a good drug experience," i.e., they increase use because they like it. Second ranked is the advice of friends, i.e., credible peers. Third ranked is drug education. Since we have found that education can serve either to facilitate expanded drug use or to restrict the spread of change, we cannot be sure whether replies to this item refer to reasons for increasing or controlling use. X and Y group members checked this item with about four times greater frequency than control group members (the greatest number, 53/506, being in the Y group). Fourth ranked is making new friends, a reply we interpret to mean new opportunities for learning about and acquiring drugs as their poor contacts expand. Fifth ranked is pressure from parents, which we presume to be primarily a restraint, although the research reminds us that children also learn to use drugs from their parents. Sixth ranked is seeing others with ill effects from drugs, a restraining form of learning. Seventh ranked is the opportunity to do things besides use drugs. A variety of other reasons were checked but responses to them were limited.

These replies suggest that, in the eyes of students, their own intimate personal and social experiences (drug experiences, friendships) are the prime factors affecting drug use change, with authoritative or institutional sources (school, parents) ranking a general second. The primary and intimate influences act, we suspect, to increase frequency, variety, and perhaps specificity of drug use and tastes, whereas the secondary authoritative and institutional sources are probably seen as restraints. It was flattering to be told that our drug education ranks foremost among the restraining forces, ahead of family, law, church, and counselors (all of which receive fewer nods on the check list), but other research data indicate that the facts are contrary, especially as regards the family. While it is very likley that youngsters in the process of expanding drug use are not fully responsive to family, church, and law, caution dictates that we treat the elevated rank of drug education here as, at best, a special sensitivity, since the youngsters were completing the questionnaire under drug education auspices; it can also express affection for their drug education teachers and passive acceptance. Had we asked nonchangers the reasons for being abstinent or stable, perhaps family, church, and law would have loomed very large. Replies, then, remind us that even under congenial teaching circumstances, students do not normally rank education as among the most salient influences on their drug use. Student awareness of influences as measured here is no proof of relative influence as might be measured objectively.

Educator Reactions

One year after our entry into the schools, an evaluation report form was given to school administrators and the regular classroom teachers of cohorts 2, 4, 6, and 8. They were asked to assess the drug education program operation, curriculum content, and observed teaching methods. We also asked them to comment on program acceptance by the students and other school personnel and we invited them to discuss any other aspect of our procedures.

Administrators commented favorably and with enthusiasm upon our work and teaching which was, they said, conducted with minimal disruption. They reported student and research staff interaction as positive and saw our teachers as well liked and having good rapport with the children. Some wanted more "progress report" meetings with the entire teaching staff.

Comments from the regular classroom teachers were very favorable. There were a few instances where teachers felt more discipline should have been used, a comment or two on room disarrangement after our sessions, and the suggestion that younger children should not be scheduled late in the day.

The administrators in town B, while commenting favorably on our staff rapport and adaptability, were unaware of our program content. This was not surprising to us since we had been asked, at program initiation, to present our objectives to the full district staff, and we were then required at the meeting to limit our presentation to fifteen minutes. This unawareness also manifested itself in the reports of the teachers. As the school superintendent observed, "Because the Stanford Drug Education Project has taken over drug education, the teachers generally tend to feel they have no responsibility in this area." Teachers were not critical of the program in any way.

Parents

We did not circulate a questionnaire to parents requesting an evaluation, but we do have data indicating parental views of drug education. First is the level of cooperation obtained at the beginning of the study, when all parents were sent forms advising them of the drug education program and giving them an opportunity to withdraw their children from the testing (but not from the teaching, which is required by law). Of 3300 parents questioned, only three disallowed their children's cooperation in the study.

During the period of our work one township, whose youngsters attended one of the high schools in which we worked, casually surveyed parents about school activities and achievements, asking them to rate the importance of drug education and asking whether or not schools were achieving parental goals in drug education. Sixty-four percent said they believed that drug education is a school responsibility; 60 percent believed it was being well achieved.

Among randomly drawn families of 235 elementary school children in the family substudy, none spontaneously voiced opposition to or disapproval of the drug education and research program we were conducting. Another assessment of parental views derives from the clinical interviews with families reported in Chapter 11. Only one of twenty-three families was opposed to the concept of education; all others favored it. In addition, during the two and one-half years of experimental teaching no parents withdrew their child from the program.

In a current project our group is conducting an experiment to see if parents are willing to become involved in the design of the drug education to be offered in the schools. Experience to date is that while parents approve that idea, very few (so far less than 3 percent of those invited) are willing to engage in planning meetings at the school.

The conclusion we reach is that the majority of our parents favor some kind of drug education. There was no opposition to the specific teaching methods or content which we relied upon. Current project experience indicates that parental interest is passive rather than active; most are not interested in being involved in curriculum planning.

Summary

Students endorse, enjoy, and say they learn from and are guided by drug education during the elementary years, especially grades 5-8, but not during high school. In all grades they liked the teachers, even when they said they were getting nothing out of what was taught. Students were most aware of learning pharmacological facts, even those in classes which were supposed to be focusing on values, decisions, and discussion. The discrepancies between what we thought we were doing and what students were sensitive to experiencing are consistent;

that stands as a warning to teachers and curriculum planners not to assume that their perceptions and those of students are the same. Students rank drug education as secondary to informal personal and social experiences as an influence on their (changing) drug use expansion, which is, as other research has shown, facilitated by these informal social influences.

With regard to their proposals for changes in our instructional approach, our students were not innovative. Insofar as they expressed themselves, they preferred more facts on drugs. The majority, even in high school, accepted whatever programs they experienced without proposals for content change. This passivity does not negate the principle of proposed major change which we infer from the fact that the majority agreed that high school was not the place to engage in drug education. It is our impression that the lack of innovation proposals and passivity may be a function of their understandable lack of experience in participating in the design of their own education. Certainly the enthusiasm which we expected for the more novel, discussion-based process education did not materialize, although some of those participating in discussion wanted more of it.

Most students appear to follow the "rational" model of education, preferring facts, acknowledging the propriety of the school's presentation of these in drug education, and conceiving of themselves as being responsive to that education—although only in elementary school years—by altering their conduct in response to the school as an influence in their lives. This readiness conforms with impact data in Chapter 6 in respect to agreement that the optimal period for intervention is in the 5th to the 8th grades. That impact data led to a more conservative appraisal of the value of drug education in elementary school than do these student evaluations. The resolution of that discrepancy is nicely summed up in the remark of one 6th grader who, on the evaluation query form, stated, "I learned a lot of things I can't remember."

School and district administrators and teachers unanimously favored our presence, work, and kinds of teacher-student interaction and presumed impact. This approval is not to be construed as universal professional interest, for in one district teachers were pleased with the project because it offered them an opportunity to do less work, and not because they utilized it as an opportunity to learn more about drug education. In this sense, the disinterest of teachers in the design and conduct of drug education is akin to the passivity existing among students.

Parents are in favor of drug education and are willing to allow their children to cooperate in evaluation programs. Parental interest does not extend, for most, to involvement in curriculum innovation. The consonance among students, teachers, and parents in their favorable views is noteworthy. So, too, is the absence of creative suggestions for change. Presumably both the approval and the absence of interest in redesign reflect confidence in the existing educational endeavor. That confidence was expressed before any evidence became available showing that drug education as we practiced it had any impact on children's drug use. This indicates either that the primary functions of drug education are not dependent upon positive impact as such, or that our consumers were more optimistic than are those of us committed to empirical evaluation. In any event we are grateful for our consumer's approval.

10 The Educational Climate

Introduction

This chapter introduces clinical observations of individual students, the expectations underlying them, and findings made in and about schools.

The primary thrust of the observations reported in this and the next two chapters is that what the individual student gets out of drug education is influenced by what he or she brings to class. Each student carries to the learning situation a unique way of experiencing himself in his own world. His or her history, abilities, and vulnerabilities greatly affect what he makes of the opportunities offered by school. Yet neither the qualities of the student nor the features of the drug education curriculum fully determine the response. The educational climate—the totality of the learning environment in school—must be reckoned with. A student's actual reaction to drug education is the product of a complex field of events; the school milieu interacts with individual personality and predilections, while many of these latter derive in turn directly from the family situation or from the neighborhood and other subcultures.

Methods in the Clinical Studies

We observed the Y and Z drug education classes in three different schools over one year. We also observed drug education in a high school which was not participating in our major study of drug education's impact, but where the teacher in one class was using our materials in the context of a social science course. In each class in the three participating schools a sample of students was interviewed. In the fourth, the nonparticipating high school, each child in class was sought out. In selecting the samples initial drug use scores as elicited on the self-report test were used to select an equal number of boys and girls from three groups; high-level users, moderate-level users, and low-level users. The grades represented were the 6th, 8th, and 11th. Twenty-three students and their families made up the final three-school sample. Thirteen students from the other high school were also seen frequently. In each case students were seen individually and were intensively interviewed. Home visits were made by the observer, accompanied by the drug education teacher, to all twenty-three homes on the three-school sample. The students own opinions and those of his parents and siblings were sought, and observations were made on family structure and interaction, discipline, emotional tone, and the role of the student in his family. With permission, the discussions were tape recorded. Later these were rated independently by the clinician and the teacher; pooled ratings were then made. At the end of the school year confidential interviews were held once again. In addition, school grades, achievement test results, teachers' notes, absenteeism records, disciplinary actions, and vice principals' observations were taken from the files to contribute added dimensions to the picture of each student's formal and informal school performance and its relationship to the home environment.

The School as Milieu

The context in which drug education takes place is the school. That is where interactions occur between the beliefs and predispositions of student, teacher, and parents insofar as parents are represented in the student's personality and opinions and in the school by its publicly determined policy.

Educational Climate in Four Schools

Two high schools—Marimba and Juniper—and two elementary schools—Watson and Harlow—offered their facilities for this study. Marimba High is an innovative school, while Juniper High is considered by students and parents to be old-fashioned; the two elementary schools are conventionally modern and serve similar communities. Marimba High, located in an all-black community, is the most unusual of the four schools.

Marimba High: A School With a Mission

It has been said by local educators of desegregated, innovative Marimba High that it is one of the best high schools in the area: "It turned a desperate educational situation into a model high school when it infused new teachers into its classrooms and attempted to desegregate the virtually all-black school." The new teachers, many of them white, are progressive. Mrs. Kinde, who teaches drug education as part of a social science course, is one of them. Principal and teachers, like many in the surrounding community, are deliberately permissive: no failing grades are given, attendance is voluntary, tardiness is not punished, and people may drift in and out of classes at will. Education is each student's personal responsbility. There is an undercurrent of two kinds of fear in the school: a general fear of violence and, on the part of teachers, a particular anxiety that students will be disapproving or disinterested. Since there is no compulsory attendance or respect, school and teachers must win over the students however they can.

Thanks to massive, repeated, district-wide recruitment efforts and offerings of a wide variety of unusual academic subjects (e.g., Hebrew, Latin, Greek, advanced calculus), the number of white students from prosperous, liberal, intellectual, middle class environments has increased considerably. At the same time, the lenient atmosphere and recreational classes (e.g., belly-dancing, African folk guitar, soul cooking) have made school tolerable to the recalcitrant truant, the academic nonachiever, the dropout, the neurotic, and the rebellious, whether black, white, or brown. Several of the best students are convinced that Marimba High has provided them with more educational opportunities than any school available in the area. They confirm that the freedom and the possibility of choosing what courses to take and how many credits is well suited to the needs of highly motivated, superior students, but is not appropriate for average students. Dull students, however, are able to fit into the program of minimal or nonexistent demands; rebellious and disinterested students survive well at Marimba, if not in the classrooms then at least out on the schoolgrounds. School itself is popular, students converge there, either to attend classes, according to their inclinations, or to hang around "where the action is"–mostly around the parking lot for the older students and in "Simba's Den" (a hamburger and ice cream stand) for the younger students.

The Nonclass. In the surrounding black neighborhoods, as in the school and reflected in the drug education class, authority, especially white authority, is unpopular. Mrs. Kinde is greatly handicapped by the prevailing enthusiasm for sabotage. At home, with her own children, Mrs. Kinde is a firm disciplinarian, a woman of solid convictions. Not so at school, for she must rely on personal charm and persuasiveness to ingratiate herself with her students. She has no authority herself or through her school administration to support her in enforcing order, civility, or attendance. The outcome, in lieu of chaos, is "permissiveness." The continuity of a regular teaching program is abandoned in favor of conversational topics dictated by the students; innumerable movies are shown during which Mrs. Kinde sometimes lies belly down on the classroom floor; she does not remonstrate with the equally relaxed, sometimes somnolent (Too much cannabis? Too many barbiturates? Too many late nights out?) conduct of her students. She does not object to the presence in class of a three-year old "cousin," or to eating and knitting, however noisy the munching and clatter. Tardiness or leaving the class elicits a saddened look, but to no avail. After several months of continuous comings and goings the disruption becomes intolerable; Mrs. Kinde locks the door. Imprisonment, the ironic and ultimate consequence of permissiveness! Not surprisingly, this too proves unacceptable. A negotiated compromise is reached: class time is reduced to half an hour of relative quiet. Attendance had always been low, and a further decline ensues. At the end of the year only three faithful students can be counted on to show up.

Class registration shows that seventeen students are enrolled, their ages varying from fourteen to eighteen years. In actual fact, no one knows who is supposed to be there. Nine was the maximum number ever present when the observer was there. An average of six students were ordinarily in class at any given moment. Students who are not present in class at all, or only for a few minutes a day, are hardly able to profit from the drug education curriculum.

Language is a compounding factor. One of those students usually present is a dull, shy, confused, Spanish-speaking youth. He will leave high school at the end of the year without reading or writing skills. He is in class because he likes Mrs. Kinde. His mental and language status prevent him from comprehending the substance of drug education. Others, Spanish speaking like the shy young man, get little out of the English language courses. True, Marimba High offers remedial English classes; of the numerous students known to need it, only one attended and soon gave it up. Without compulsion or motivation the classroom is empty. The black dialect is hard for Mrs. Kinde (or the observing clinician) to understand. We both wonder how much black students (a theoretical thirteen out of seventeen) can learn from teachers whose English must seem just as incomprehendible.

Drug Education. Mrs. Kinde had planned to teach our Stanford drug curriculum within the context of her social studies program, renamed "group dynamics" to render it more appealing to students. Since Mrs. Kinde's well-founded fears are that her students might desert her should the subject matter prove disagreeable or boring, she seldom finds an opportune time to say anything at all about drugs. The luring of students to attend has first priority. Mrs. Kinde, therefore, runs the movie machine. It is up to the observer-clinician to introduce drug-related subjects whenever possible, which is not often.

Individual interviews with each student had been planned, and later, for all of the families. This proves to be impossible. Mrs. Kinde hesitates to tell her students about the project; she doubts they will cooperate. She is right; it is difficult to corral most of them for even a five-minute chat, let alone for a serious discussion or a home visit. Appointments are made; they are not kept. A tour of the school grounds locates one girl in a fistfight with her boyfriend, another playing basketball, a few are busy grooming each other's hair, others claim urgent appointments or cannot be found. Only the rare student is in a mood to talk.

Marimba: A Conclusion. Here at Marimba one learns that to call a place a school does not make it one. There can be no learning if there is no attendance. If there is attendance there will be no learning of planned substance if the course content is not presented. Even if it is presented there will be no learning if the class is in chaos, if children do not comprehend what is said, if there is no attentive respect, or if the real "business" of teachers and students centers on other things: being afraid, gaining approval, minding the baby, derogating authority, eating, or sleeping off fatigue or some drug effect. Marimba is both an experiment and a social reality; it is not a place where drug education in the classroom (we do not speak of the parking lot and the rest rooms) takes place, no matter what the formal agenda may claim.

Juniper High: Old-fashioned

The traditional, coercive environment at Juniper High and the conventionality of the two elementary schools permitted the interview phase of our study to go forward. While not all of the students were always present in the drug education classes—as explained below—they, unlike the Marimba students, nevertheless took the drug tests. All of them cooperated with the personal interviews, and their parents cooperated in the at-home discussions.

No one claims that students come to Juniper with enthusiasm; school here is not like Marimba, "where the action is." They come because they must: parents and truant officers see to that. The atmosphere is a bit gloomy; the buildings are in large renaissance mission style; the grounds, although attractive, are not the place for informal group conviviality; and the school is patrolled by husky aides hired to prevent trouble. Juniper has had its share of turbulence in the past. Now the corridors are almost deserted during class time; the class-cutting student will find his colleagues outside the school building, not in the corridors. There is none of the relaxed, jolly or frightful, intense social life of Marimba.

The Students and the Community. Juniper is a much larger school than Marimba. Its students are from multiethnic backgrounds. Many come from Spanish, Mexican, and Italian families, with a sprinkling of Greek and Portuguese. The majority is white, the minority is black.

The population served by the Juniper High School district is much more stable than that of the Marimba community. Many of the students' parents have themselves attended the school in their time.

Unlike what the police records tell us for Marimba's locale, the adult community in the Juniper district is largely law abiding, insists on being well served, and is protected by its police force. Juniper High reflects this only in part, for while most regulations and rules are enforced in traditional authoritarian ways, this does not prevent a good deal of interracial friction and straightforward hoodlumism. Racial strife is reported to be on the decline, but not theft, vandalism, and fights. Much unsightly littering is evident. Cars are apparently a favorite target for breakins. Classes are large, quiet, and disciplined. Corridor life surges only fiercely and noisily between class periods. But here, too, many students are afraid.

The Drug Education Class. At Juniper our regular drug education classes proceed on schedule. They are taught by our teams during P.E. periods.

Attendance, however, is very poor, in spite of its being "mandatory." The problem is that the drug education class time competes with the P.E. program. Although drug education is a required subject, administrator planning and follow-through were inadequate. The P.E. teachers were supposedly instructed to send students to the drug education classes and to record absences for those failing to do so. Teachers, in fact, often allow them to stay in P.E.—a more important subject in both P.E. teachers' and students' opinions—or to leave. There is no way to insure or monitor drug class attendance. Students, of course, cannot learn in a class from which they are absent.

Juniper: A Conclusion. At Juniper, we have learned that administrative competence and teacher cooperation are needed to ensure that rules and actualities are the same.

Watson and Harlow: Two Modern Elementary Schools

The harmony among school and community, teachers and students, is striking in these two small, handsome, modern elementary schools with neatly kept, spacious, orderly playgrounds. Both schools are situated in well-to-do, middle class, white neighborhoods; classes are small and informal, yet well run; students and teachers are at ease. They smile and greet each other. Newcomers are welcomed and made to feel at home. Here, as at Juniper High, our team teaches the drug education classes. Unlike Juniper, roll is carefully taken. If a student is absent, he must have a valid excuse or his parents are called. Attendance at the drug education classes reflects the general excellent record keeping.

Unlike the high school counselors at Juniper and Marimba, the Vice Principals at the elementary schools make it their business to know the teachers and students well. They assess them sympathetically and realistically and handle conflict with great good sense and to excellent effect. They also know their students' home situations; they are aware of the extent to which this affects the learning endeavor.

Of great importance to our drug program is the administrative interest in its success. Not only do the Vice Principals keep track of each class and who teaches it, but also help resolve conflicts should they arise. They personally assist in getting students out of class for interviews and give liberally of their own time to share their knowledge about individual students. The conditions under which the drug education program proceeds are optimal, as are the conditions for teaching in general. The students' attitudes toward their schools reflect this: they like their school; a troublemaker, even if suspended, will return to the schoolgrounds, only to be sent home again in vain. He is afraid of being bored if not in school.

Watson and Harlow: A Conclusion. The conclusion is in the description. Drug education can proceed as a pedagogical fact when it is in harmony with community interest, when students concur in acting as they are "supposed to," and in the presence of administrative support and competence.

The Student Backgrounds

Two quite divergent student populations attend Marimba High; one is from the immediate black neighborhood, mostly from working class families, many with parents on welfare. There are recent immigrants from the south. There is a great deal of separation, divorce, and illegitimacy in one section of town. Yet many people are related to each other. The black students have innumerable aunts, uncles, and cousins, real or contrived. They feel at home locally, resist efforts to "sneak them out" or be bused into the more distant, cold, and formal white school systems. The community divides itself into the "Christians" and "the others." Among the latter, unemployment is rampant, as is crime. Their children engage in vandalism, delinquency, alcohol, and violence.

White students attending Marimba from distant well-to-do communities are tolerated without noticeable racial incidents. They do segregate themselves from blacks that "hang around" or attend predominantly recreational classes. The whites take academic subjects; each group keeps apart on the schoolgrounds. The white students at Marimba High are from predominantly liberal intellectual families; they live in orderly, well-protected, safe neighborhoods. At home, permissiveness and personal explorations are encouraged, as is academic achievement and economic success. In consequence, as we have seen in our other work (Blum and Associates, 1973), both their drug use scores and their school grades are high.

The children attending Watson and Harlow Elementary are from less-affluent and more solidly middle class and conventional families than those who encourage their children to embark on the adventures of Marimba High. There is little divorce; all families but one we saw are white; one is of third-generation Italian stock, another is first-generation German. The only black student is from a prosperous, professional family. Their conduct in school and with drugs is conventional.

Juniper High students in our sample are also relatively homogeneous. All are from North European families, with the exception of one third-generation Italian family. All fathers are employed in trades. Over half the students are living with their biological parents in intact, comfortable, lower middle class homes. The consequences of socioeconomic background for educational achievement are too well known to be repeated here.

We do vividly see that differences in class attendance symbolize the gulf that separates the academically motivated, conscientiously attending, disciplined students who come from affluent families and the poor, unmotivated, often delinquent, truancy-prone students. The drug use patterns of the latter, though perhaps no different in degree, are not amenable to educational modification, since they do not voluntarily expose themselves to it; nor are they receptive should class attendance be enforced. As we saw at Juniper, there needs to be administrative and teacher control to be sure that the middle group of students, those academically disinterested but conformingly responsive to authority, will attend class. Such enforced attendance does not guarantee interest or learning, but is an initial requirement for any formal teaching. In such instances, as the World Health Association has noted, "teaching" may be quite different from "education."

11 Parental Influence and Children's Responses

Introduction

In this chapter observations are presented which derive from interviews with parents and their children. Its thrust is to show that the reaction of the child to drug education reflects his experiences at home. The observations suggest, not incidentally, that the school's drug education itself reflects family influences as to how children are to be guided and toward what ends.

Beliefs About Drug Education

The conceptual climate in which drug education is embedded is comprised of the expectations of and attitudes toward drug education on the part of teachers, parents, and students. Students' views are frequently the internalized reflection of what their parents think and of what they sometimes say. This inner geography of belief, prejudice, and expectation becomes a codeterminant of what the student hears or chooses not to hear in class; it is one of the forces that shape his learning.

Educators give at least lip service to the presumed utility of providing drug education in school, regardless of how qualified their staffs may be. No one we met questioned it, so certain are they all of a positive outcome. With the exception of Marimba, the schools reflect the hopes of the community as seen through the eyes of the parents. The parents we saw unanimously support drug education in the schools, although a few may voice an occasional stricture. The philosophy of our study group's drug education teachers closely resembles that of the parents and schools. Our teachers are devoted, convinced that what they do has intrinsic value. Insofar as students do not profit, it is not because the staff lacked enthusiasm or, as we could see in class, commitment to the curriculum.

Given the remarkable congruity of belief among community educators and parents (and contrary to this observer's own deep skepticism), it would be astonishing if the children, at least the younger ones, were to disagree. There need be no astonishment, for they do not. What they do in secret is another matter; and also quite a different matter will be their drug use as adults. Below we present a few quotes to illustrate why parents and students believe that drug education is a "good thing."

Why Drug Education is Good

Some of the positive remarks from students at Juniper High reveal that drug education is useful in evading more difficult classes, like physics. Parents are more often vague about its merits: "It is good in any case," says Isabella's mother, "regardless whether it is useful in changing drug use and risk taking." She hopes very sincerely that drug education in school will continue: "it would be the biggest mistake in the whole world if they ever dropped it. I don't think parents can ever do a good enough job; school has to help."

She tells us clearly what many other parents imply: school is the ally of the home and its function is to complement the parental effort at socializing the child. It is a socialization for the whole community. Parents are optimistic that the school can take children from diverse social, ethnic, and economic backgrounds and mold them into an adult community with consensus on what is important and how one should behave. The school is to provide the ammunition for parents to turn their own children into good citizens, and they expect the school to do the same for other peoples' children. The goal is unspoken but very important: the creation of a community which can coexist by sharing the same expectations.

Yet the school can serve this cementing and unifying function only if there is already basic agreement among children, parents, and school authorities that presiding over the melting pot *is* one of its functions. At Marimba this cannot take place for there is no agreement, overt or covert, on a common goal and on the importance of community mutuality in child rearing. Marimba represents not simply diversity or pluralism but a defensive subcommunity resisting penetration through teaching. Describing the two situations, the one encouraging conformity, the other confirming de facto separateness, does not imply that one is better than the other. There are arguments in favor of both diversity and likeness.

Do Parents Have a Teaching Role?

To hear them tell, one would not ascribe any drug guidance to parents. Parents, school, and children seem to share the notion, a peculiar one we believe, that the educator, as a professional, and however untrained for the specific job, is the only one who can effectively educate students to sensible drug use. Over and over, the observer hears confessions of incompetence on the part of parents. Few of their children disagree with them, although, judging by the results, we believe most do a splendid job of child rearing. We cite a few examples.

A Genteel Autocratic Household

Gretchen, like many children, believes that parents do not know much about drugs. She is a well behaved, almost priggish, 6th grader at Watson Elementary school, who would not dare to demonstrate anything but model behavior when it comes to drugs. She likes drug education, for "it's still good to learn [about it] in school because parents don't know as much as you [teacher] could teach us." Her family holds a tight rein; father exerts a soft-spoken, quiet authority that brooks no questioning. Mother, more vivacious, is aware that the iron fist is most effective when it wears a velvet glove. She says, with an appearance of tolerance, that she wants: "The kids to turn out what they want to be, as long as they are satisfied with themselves. As long as they respect the laws, whatever they may be." The theme of unquestioning obedience dressed up as the children's best interest pervades the household. Mother's philosophy is to rear the children so "they can make their own decisions, but catch them so young that it will be the right one." Could Gretchen possibly decide to use drugs even if her teachers were to tell her that alcohol and marijuana are used safely by most people? Or if a girlfriend tried to persuade her to take a "pill" for fun? Hardly, for this family has "absolutely no use for drugs, whatever they are. We don't drink anything in this house. I stay away from smoking people; I stay away from drinking people; they have nothing to say to me . . . this is no way of living." Mother does not think she is expert enough to teach about drugs, but her rejection of people who use drugs is so calmly final that it makes a deep impression. She lets her children know where they would stand with her "*If. . . .*" What can school add to such effective teaching?

Self-confident though he is, Gretchen's father agrees with his daughter that school can do far more than he is able to. It can "teach them so they are protected against pushers." Other parents, less sure of themselves, rely heavily and hopefully on school, with their children's explicit concurrence.

The Addiction-Prone Household

Huck's mother is the most extreme in her appeal for help from school. Neither she nor his father consider themselves fit to convey the "dos" and "don'ts" about drugs. Both say that they are addicted, the father to alcohol, as was his father, the mother to cigarettes and coffee. The mother says: "My kids come home from school and give it to me: they say 'don't smoke,' and I have to tell them: 'I'm weak, I can't stop' . . . they [cigarettes] control my life . . . I don't have the right to say to them 'You are not to smoke.' " Her husband agrees completely with her; he feels that he cannot forbid the children to drink since he himself may "feel remorseful the next day; it'll last for a day or a week; but anyway when I have been wrong [drunk] I know I have been and I try to atone in certain ways of my own . . . but to sit down and talk!" This he cannot do. He is sure he must leave the drug talk to the school. Huck's parents do not realize that they are far more effective and potent teachers than school can ever hope to be.

In this subsample, there are three alcoholic fathers and several alcoholic grandfathers whose children and some of their grandchildren are *all* ardent teetotalers. Huck's father explains: "I would think that all three of my boys have seen me with too much and I think it has leaned them in the other direction where we can't even get them to have a little glass of wine at Thanksgiving for the simple reason that they have seen Dad when he had too much." His sons and others with alcoholic fathers confirm this: "[I've seen him] drunk ... and you don't want to be like that." Can school teach more? Astonishingly, Huck's mother credits the school: "We have three boys and it's to the credit of the school that they are not on drugs." Neither parent appreciates what the father has accomplished by his honesty, his simple, convincing, firm explanations, and his obvious love for his boys. Nor does the mother acknowledge her own efforts in directing the boys along the straight and narrow path. She thinks that she is incapable and helpless, as do so very many mothers to whom we have talked (see Blum and Associates, 1972a). Actually, they have a far greater impact on the actual behavior than does the school.

Huck's mother's protestations of ignorance overlook the fact that she knows very well what she wants to achieve and what she wants the school to teach: "I have three boys, and I don't even know what they are talking about; grass is the only word I know what it means." His mother believes that Huck is expert on drugs. Is he? Not at all. He has tried to smoke cigarettes but gave them up; he has had some beer, wine, and occasionally a little liquor (his father asks him to be his "bartender"), but has had no other drugs. Huck's mind is made up not to use them. He does not credit the school for his resolution; he says he decided on this course of action before he ever had drug education. His parents' not wanting him to smoke helped him to quit. They do not know that.

A Family in Need of Help

Judy's parents feel hopelessly inadequate to teach about drugs; they too would like the school to do the job. They are confused, and well they might be, by what their children tell them about the drug world in which they live. Judy's mother complains: "My children laugh at me. I don't know that much about it. We never had much education that way and our children are far more educated on those two subjects [dope and VD] than we ever were." Judy tortures her mother with ridicule and with her own extreme conduct. Judy, age 17, has used all of the drugs on our list except heroin. She overeats, has had an intimate relationship with a boy now in prison, she is vividly dramatic, and worse, she is genuinely forgetful, confused, and afraid. "If I didn't have my friends, I'd go crazy," she warns.

And what does Judy think of drug education? It is to the good, she says, because "it got me out of physical education." Does she remember anything of what was taught? That would be impossible; she confesses that she did not go to the class. She is an habitual truant and cannot stand school. She exclaims in an exaggerated, tragic-comic sing-song: "I don't think I can *take* school that much more: *twelve years* . . . I struggle. . . ." She ends on an unexpected, inappropriate giggle. She adds that it was her mother's insistence that induced her to stop smoking; certainly school had nothing to do with it, nor even her friends. She is explicit on that point, a point of extraordinary importance.

Judy, the most disturbed child in the subsample, the one who ranks highest in drug use, is amenable to parental discipline, however impervious she may be to other influences and however discouraged and inadequate her mother is made to feel. It is this mother who, *if* she persists and survives, will be the one most likely to guide the troubled spirit of her child into safe harbors. The word "survival" is used purposely. Judy's mother has high blood pressure, is very excitable, and becomes inordinately depressed on the tranquilizers her physician has prescribed. She is concerned about dying; perhaps this is an exaggeration of her actual physical state, but also is, no doubt, an attempt to convey her need for assistance. This family sorely needs help. Their thought that school offers reinforcement of parental standards for behavior is a consolation to them, a ray of hope. That Judy does not bother to come to class matters less, since the very fact that the class is there, that the school considers it important, strengthens the parental position.

The parents that we talked to represent a continuum of skill and success in shaping their children's attitudes and behavior along socially approved lines, from those with a firm and loving approach to those who vacillate and fear to displease their children lest they lose their love. All of them, however, give their approval to drug education—whatever it may be, whatever good it may do—because it gives them support in their own battle to civilize and safeguard their children.

What Students Hear

The Voice of Conscience

Parental feelings of inadequacy notwithstanding, their children hear very well what they are told, however disguised the message. More than that, interviews with the students show that what they believe their parents want them to learn is what they believe their teacher is telling them. Each student in our subsample was asked what he thought the drug education teacher was trying to get across to him. Since we also observed the teaching, it became evident that what the students imagine the teacher says has little to do with what she does say. They only hear one message, a simple one: "Don't use drugs." They hear this message long before the teacher has opened her mouth. At Marimba, the brightest students agree that drug education is a waste of time since they know what the teacher will say, regardless. The teacher is clearly the mouthpiece of their consciences, the spoken or implicit voice of their parents. In all four of the schools, at all class levels and achievement levels, students believe that the schools must have the same aims as their parents. Our program had not envisaged itself in this way, but nevertheless that is how it is perceived. The students were better sociologists than we.

The Voice of Reason

Some children elaborate on this theme: "Mom says not to use it; school tells me why not." Pretty little Alice, an 8th grader who always cooperates, puts it concisely: "You teach us all the dangers and we make up our minds." Her mother confirms this: "Let the kids decide for themselves not to use; give them the facts so they can come to the right decision." Alice elaborates the point: "Before drug education I didn't think I'd take drugs, now I know I won't." Gretchen holds a like view of the matter: "Well, I think you probably want me to make my own decision, but you probably want me to know how it's dangerous and all that." (Both girls are in the Z program practicing value clarification and decision making.) Orson thinks drug education is "pretty good, it tells me how dangerous drugs are." He is in the didactic Y program. Frankie reports the same: "I think it's good, convinces us that we shouldn't use things that are harmful—cigarettes, drugs, drink."

Subtle Coercion

School, parents, and children agree on another point: how to convince the child by allowing him to come to his own conclusions and to make the *right* decision. Making up one's own mind is a frequent theme. Throughout the family discussions, allowing children opportunity to decide freely is heard again and again. These remarks do not reflect permissiveness nor a wish for the child to reach reasoned decisions, for while the child is supposed to believe that he has decided on a course of action quite on his own it must be one that is morally acceptable. One of the older students has clearly adopted the method for herself. She will, so she says, rear her own children by "a combination of all the facts, telling them what I think, exposing them to both sides; I hope they decide the right way." She sounds like her own mother talking. For that matter, is not that the real aim of the community and the school, and of our decision making and didactic classes as well?

As one listens to those parents who have had the most success in their child rearing, one notes that the same method is applied to the whole range of conduct requiring socialization. Give the children a long rein, let them think that they are independent, give them information, allow them to elect their own course, but make sure that they are hedged in by subtle guidelines all along the way. The canny children, the rebellious ones, those whose parents have shown their hands, can see what the game is. If they are loving and obedient, they go along. The game is mutually respectful and has the ring of democracy to it, but whatever the ploy, they want to be what their parents desire. Others will pay lip service but will go their own way. The latter will have made their own conforming decisions, much to the annoyance of school and parents. For those Marimba students whose life style is already far different from that of the surrounding world, it is easier to recognize the stranger's squeeze play and to be suspicious of sugared words. Their suspicions keep them far enough away so as not to be enticed.

Science and Facts

What propaganda can be more subtle than that based on impersonal and noncontroversial fact? Scientific data are acceptable to consumer and producer alike. A child can hardly elect to rebel against objective reality as readily as he might against subjective morality. And so we find that families, school, and students are agreed on yet another point, the desirability of providing technical information on drugs. Parents expect school to bolster their implicit or explicit prohibition with the "scientific data" they themselves feel they lack. They are preconvinced that the data are compatible with their beliefs, and their children and their children's teachers believe that it is not enough in an age of reason to invoke morality by itself as a guiding principle. Such guidance is made credible by higher authority: twentieth century American science. "Give them the facts," demand the parents. They mean: "Tell the dangers," and "No need to tell them what alcohol is good for . . . tell them about the harm alcohol does."

When parents say they want the school to give the "facts," to provide a scientific halo for their own moral teaching at home, the "facts" they expect are those of the bad effects. The teachers echo: "We are not here to preach"; yet that is what their students expect them to do and, as we have seen, are firmly convinced they do. Nevertheless, they too would like to hear some facts, but perhaps not for the same purposes as their parents.

Clarity, Not Confusion

Sandy has a hippie mother whose ex-junkie boyfriend lives with them. Sandy knows that "they don't want me to use any drugs," although his mother does not have the courage to tell him that outright. Sandy's home has been the scene of frightening experiences, of family friends spending time in drug trances, breaking furniture, acting "weirdly," and passing out. Sometimes Sandy has nightmares. He gets "mixed up" when he sees, hears, or reads something "scary." He likes drug education "the way it is taught." It serves a double function for him; on the one hand, it says openly what his mother dare not say out loud for fear he would do the opposite, and on the other hand it helps him understand the otherwise incomprehensible drug-induced behavior on the part of his parents' friends. Those facts do not change the nature of his house, but they help Sandy keep his nightmares and fantasies under control. For the sake of Sandy's mental health those facts objectify and somewhat neutralize the awful things he sees.

Pragmatic Considerations

There is another type of student who wishes to hear "facts" about drugs. He is the one who already knows a great deal about their effects from personal acquaintance. He has tried a good many drugs and plans to continue using them, but he is worried that he might come to harm. How much is safe? "I'd like to know, so I would take the right amount and not get killed." "It's important to know the names [of drugs] if you need them," (to buy illicitly) is Dennis' opinion. Articulate Katy, an outstanding black athlete much admired for getting drunk and "staying cool" at the same time, speaks for many when she emphasizes the importance of money, but she is one of the few who understand the role of school in preparing one to obtain it. For her, school is the place that will help her to get a job, "So one can earn money [legitimately] to buy drugs, instead of having to steal and rob."

Facts for Facts' Sake

A different type of student is one who loves to learn, comes to school prepared from home to enjoy acquiring new knowledge and skills. This student is equally as enthusiastic about receiving drug information as any other schooling. Approval of drug classes is frequently expressed in the same breath as a liking for most school subjects.

Other Actions

Taboo and Curiosity

The maxims "Catch them young" and "Scare them away from drugs" work for awhile. What happens to the occasional student so thoroughly indoctrinated and strictly reared when the attitudes learned at home are at variance with those expressed by his drug education teacher? Perry's case is an example. His parents fully support the drug education program; they view drugs with great alarm and have inculcated their forebodings in their offspring; his father even worries that some teachers might be too permissive or possibly smoke "pot" themselves. An unmodulated disciplinarian, he runs the family as an old-fashioned autocrat. His son Perry is a tall, smiling, self-possessed, friendly 11th grader at Juniper. He earns good money and has managed to become independent in spite of his father's dominating manner. What has drug education meant to him? He found it helpful in emancipating himself from his family. Drug education has made him aware that drugs "are around more than you think; it makes them more acceptable." It also made him "somewhat more curious" about drugs. His interest aroused and reassured by what he had been taught, Perry has gone out to test the matter for himself. He now smokes marijuana often.

Restrictively reared children use the relatively greater permissiveness of views expressed in drug education classes to shed the taboos they bring with them from their homes.

A number of parents in our sample rightly anticipate such an outcome. They worry lest drug education might arouse curiosity—as indeed it has in Perry's case—and stir up a hornet's nest—which it has not. One father, himself veering toward alcoholism, cautions: "What you don't know, don't heat you up." Another father, though confident that he can trust school to teach and his son to learn how to make the right decisions with regard to drugs, admonishes: "[curiosity], that's one thing we don't have to encourage. Curiosity, that's natural, and may lead the kids on."

Self-reliance and Independent Judgment

Isabella's parents are unlike Perry's; they do not fear experimentation. They believe a child must be allowed to make errors in order to learn. Her father may "steer" but will never "push." Isabella is a free and jolly spirit, allowed to go her own way, secure in the knowledge that she will not be allowed to go too far. Her family, of Italian background, encourages her to taste wine with meals. Her ideas are received with respect. Her parents have taught her to expect helpful information from school which she is to evaluate according to its merits. For an 8th grader she is exceptionally mature; she too realizes that teachers "try to teach you, try to influence you not to take [drugs] ... try to scare you away from it reasonably." She does make up her mind about drugs, just as she has been encouraged to by her parents in other matters of conduct, but it occurs within the secure framework of family example and teaching and her already sensible judgment. Isabella is in a position to evaluate the drug education course itself. She can do that rationally because her family and her maturity have made her a reasonable person. In talking to Isabella we are reminded that some youngsters are more mature in regard to drug matters than their teachers.

12 Reactions in the Classroom

Certain characteristics of children occur frequently enough and are sufficiently salient to make them important in understanding classroom reactions to drug education materials. This chapter identifies such characteristics as observed during clinical interviews or in classrooms. Suggestions are offered as to what might be done about some of those features which reduce the impact of drug education.

Student Characteristics

Being Turned Off

Surfeit is one of the most pernicious factors that "turn the kids off." Many of the students at Marimba, and perhaps at other schools as well, spend inordinate amounts of time at home viewing TV. Mrs. Kinde's "terrible trio," the fourteen-year old chatterboxes, sometimes stay up until 2 A.M. or even 4 A.M. watching horror movies. Is it any wonder that they are inattentive when they are presented with yet another of the innumerable films which are ground out by the Marimba projectors, hour after hour, class after class?

Evaluations of films by the class immediately after viewing indicates that most students do not in any event understand what drug education movies are about. Only three out of fourteen students present comprehend what the *National Drinking Game* (admittedly aimed at a more adult audience) tries to convey. Of these three, only one really comes close. Another film, *Mind-Benders*, a special school-age film, is lost on them because none can remember seeing an essential sequence portraying the potential risks of genetic damage due to drug use. They are unable to recall even simple scenes such as the mice sitting in cages waiting for drug injections.

The least-difficult film, one in which only two actors appear as mother and daughter, is better remembered. When urged to reflect on what they have seen, it turns out that the students misinterpret it, consonant with their inner preoccupations. "Don't get high on drugs because there might be no one to help you if you get in trouble," is what one girl believes this film is about. Another, himself afraid he will be placed into a class for the retarded, thinks that the heroine is mentally retarded. One student concludes with satisfaction, "Grown-ups is just as worse as kids; they no better than anyone else." For the objective observer of the film the message was about a mother-daughter conflict.

161

We doubt the efficacy of movies that are untested. Why not require of any drug education film that it be pretested by the maker, using scientific sampling to identify the age, drug experience, and intellectual capabilities of the audiences for whom it is suited? The procedure, in essence, is the same as that used for prescription information to physicians describing indications and side effects. The Federal Trade Commission could supervise truth in such packaging.

The Medium is the Wrong Message

Why are many of the students in Mrs. Kinde's class so particularly lacking in understanding, so recalcitrant? We are aware that there has been much speculation on the lack of fit between conventional (upper, middle, and working class) values as represented by schools and the interests of black, urban, and disadvantaged youngsters. Our remarks are limited to what we saw, heard, and now interpret.

The rejection of drug education, like most other "normal" courses at Marimba, is active, not simply passive. Talking, moving about, eating, falling asleep, interrupting–these and other activities do not simply represent a style of living, they have a function in the class. The function is the same one found in being absent. It is to avoid listening, to avoid the message. Mrs. Kinde puts it this way: "Someone is out to sell them something and they're doing their level best not to buy." That implies that if they were to hear the message they would respond and that they are defending against that possibility. One surmises a fear that the message can capture them and that it must be avoided completely, rather than heard and then utilized advantageously for their own purposes, whatever these might be. The black students in class were, it seems, resisting the "white imperative" lest it encroach on them and present them with dilemmas they would rather avoid.

What is the message? In drug education or elsewhere it can be achievement, discipline, competition, future orientation, interpersonal distance, pleasure-avoidance, lawfulness, and work. Contrast that with the day-to-day lives at Marimba: intensely sociable, active fun, concrete, dramatic, and immediate. Why should a student want to trade the latter for the former? If a student opens himself to the lure of the achieving, abstemious future he must reject the present and not only change but also aspire. And in aspiring there is risk of failure, failure because the system is foreign, because it is difficult, and because one is unprepared; and one's friends cannot help because they are also unprepared.

Boredom

Students in schools besides Marimba High have also not learned to learn. They loathe sitting still in class, prefer athletics to the multiplication table, and want their days filled with excitement. They want the school to show "gory movies" for a thrill, and they suggest, slyly, that our drug educators bring real drugs to class so they may see "what they look like." Privately they say this would be a good opportunity to "rip them off." These students are bored, and there is nothing a traditional school can do about it. What about early school leaving at age fourteen and vocational education?

Sensitivity

It would not do to select more dramatic films to arouse the perennially bored student. In the younger grades and among many of the girls, blood and gore evokes only a negative reaction. We find that the student who genuinely feels sensitivity for others comes out of the drug education classes depressed when the discussions or films highlight the sorry antecedents and consequences of drug abuse. He tries his best to forget (repress) the whole thing. Sensitive people need a gentle education.

"I don't like to see gross pictures," says another. He is not actually thinking of the films he has seen in our program, but rather those shown in driver safety education, but it is all the same to him. He does not want to endure the sight of "chopped-off heads." A number of the girls are upset by the same idea and dislike drug films in which they must look at hypodermic syringes or strung-out junkies. This generation of students reared on TV violence are presumed to be inured to anything. Not all of them are; perhaps this is a good sign.

Critical Developmental Periods

A number of boys between ten and twelve express a fear of dying. Not only the students who use excessive amounts of dangerous drugs worry about it, but also some of those in the lower-use group associate drugs with death. They seem to be at an age where they are particularly vulnerable to fears of death (in psychodynamic terms one would speak of castration fears coming to the surface). Consequently, the boys who are involved in drugs are disappointed if drug education "fails" them. By that they mean that they have not been taught how much they may safely take without risking an overdose, or what drugs they can safely mix together. They want technical advice on drug use, but their wish is founded deep in fears typical of their age. Ordinary education cannot easily cope with such psychodynamics.

Vocabulary

Not many students admit that the drug vocabulary is beyond their ability to understand. Bright and motivated students are seen in the library checking out the unfamiliar technical terms. For the rest, much that is taught simply passes over their heads. The drug educator dare not assume too much about student knowledge.

Physiological Inattentiveness

At Marimba, one boy in class was hungry. One day when we talked he said he would have his first and only meal after school, one that he would prepare himself. One suspects that his parents are wetbacks—illegal immigrants—without work and afraid to apply for welfare or food stamps. When the boy is hungry he is weak and inattentive; his brain fails him, his stomach preoccupies him.

Much more often the students arrive in class high, low, or hung over, all drug responses. Many are simply and prosaically tuckered out. Jessica tells of partying and boozing all night. The shy fellow staring out of the window before he drops to sleep has been tagging after his older brothers, "rowdy dudes" who stay up much of the night. Night is a busy time for Marimba's people; the day is for fraternizing and catching up on sleep. There is no time for education.

Age

The older students have long since made up their minds with regard to drug use and are firmly entrenched in their ways or waywardness. Drug education for many at Juniper and Marimba high schools, like academic education in general, is seen as irrelevant to student life goals. Those from working class families are intent on getting out of school, learning a trade, and earning good wages. The patterns of cigarette smoking, beer on the job, and drinks after work are part of the family and vocational pattern; students are already well into it.

Middle and upper class youngsters are also, by high school age, committed to enacting the customs of their families and the other groups of which all are a part; religious, political, and vocational. They are, essentially, adult in their drug habits, although, as with other adolescent uncertainty and impulsiveness, they are not as consistent or as careful as adults. This explains the deaths from speeding and drunken driving at Juniper during the year of observation. One student had to be removed from the school grounds by ambulance; he had taken an overdose and was discovered unconscious in the bushes. No doubt other such mishaps occurred.

The few older students who are emotionally unstable are engaged in deviant drug use. They are, if not already in visible trouble, rapidly headed in that direction. Their families lost control some time ago and the child qua student, now truant or a dropout, will not be reached by his teachers any more than by his parents. Hospitals or jails will see him finally; drug education will have made no difference.

But One Stroke for Many Folks

We reviewed both the scores on the Thorndike-Lorge word mastery test (verbal intelligence) and the grades and attendance records from the files of the seventeen youths in Mrs. Kinde's class. The two Marimba groups described in Chapter 10—aspiring, academically oriented whites, and local, educationally poorly performing blacks—were reflected in class score distributions. On all measures the two groups were entirely separate. The self-selected gifted whites are hands down favorites over the academically handicapped or message-rejecting blacks.

Consider, for example, the two best students in Mrs. Kinde's class. One girl is a National Merit Scholar; both girls have been accepted by fine colleges. Both score brilliantly in verbal intelligence, attend class diligently, and get high grades. And neither uses any of the unsanctioned drugs or plans to in the future. Compare this with the others, where our estimate of high drug use is substantiated by Katy, an admired but often drunk girl: "Half [of my black friends] come to school loaded, drunk, or high."

Consider now the composition of students in Mrs. Kinde's class, the diversity of socioeconomic background, age, attendance, motivation, drug experience, intellectual ability, delinquency, resistance, inattentiveness, and sensitivity. Each child is, of course, unique; nevertheless they can be roughly grouped by shared traits. How many subgroups are there among the sometimes seventeen students in this class? Certainly the two subgroups black and white, as noted above, and the subgroups "rowdies" and "Christians;" undoubtedly there are more than that as well. How can Mrs. Kinde proceed with a single format for drug education and ever hope to reach these immensely different audiences? Indeed, with any format available to her, how many could she reach?

Aptitude and Teaching Methods

A portion of the students in the *Z* program fail to see how discussions about other peoples' problems have anything to do with drug education. It is "not relevant," is "a waste of time," or "We haven't talked about drugs yet and the year is just about up." Some are disappointed and indignant. They want facts, scientific data, figures, and concrete examples. However, not everybody reacts this way to the *Z* program. A clear difference exists between those who reject the *Z* program and those who like it.

Those in the subsample who are mechanically inclined, who enjoy manipulative, object-related activities, who prefer spelling and grammar over reading novels, are also the ones who favor the didactic *Y* program and complain about the irrelevancies of the *Z* process program. The students who are oriented toward people, who plan to go into nursing and social work, who like drama and story writing but dislike spelling and grammar, feel that the *Z* discussion classes are interesting and allow them to come to grips with their own decisions. This difference between "objective" interests and "personal" interests is maintained beyond puberty; it is found at the high school level as well as at the elementary level. The subsample is too small to permit generalization. However, it does suggest that differences in interests and orientation may be associated with differing affinities for the Y and Z approaches.

The Z Program in the Schools

The assumption in developing process education was that it is good to bring problems out in the open, discuss them, recognize them for what they are, and, it is hoped, do something constructive as a result. Is the classroom the place for openness? Should it be? Is it the place where constructive action can be taken? On the basis of what the students themselves say this assumption is dubious. Younger and older students agree that it is very hard to talk about one's difficulties in class. Shyness is the first obstacle, but after a little while that could be overcome, they think. The next obstacle is that their schoolmates are not to be trusted. How can one depend on those others not "ratting" to the Principal? In the younger grades, maintaining "face" is the first and most absorbing task of the youngsters. A harmless remark—to an adult—such as liking a certain girl, can bring on blushes of deep shame and the laughter of derision. There are delicacies and pitfalls which spell quick doom for a "group dynamics" discussion in the ordinary classroom. There is, after all, no unifying purpose and communality of interest at stake. School is not group psychotherapy, and should not be. In contrast, the informal didactic Y programs are more successful and harmless. Discussion and evaluation can always be incorporated in any didactic program without asking students to make unnecessary, self-damaging revelations. The additional advantage of the didactic approach is that it does not demand skills which an ordinary teacher does not already possess.

Summing Up Chapters 10, 11, and 12

Observations were made in two elementary and two high schools. Six classrooms were the scenes of observations over a one-year period. Thirty-six students were interviewed, as were twenty-three of their families. Objective data on all these students were also obtained, including grades, school attendance, and, for twenty-three in the main subsample, their drug use scores. The methods were those of the clinical psychologist acting as a participant observer.

The quality of and response to drug education is immensely affected by the community milieu, and the school is the reflection of that milieu. If the school is there not primarily to teach but to serve other community purposes, drug education will not be taught, regardless of what claims may be made. If the students do not attend class, or if they attend but are defensive, indifferent, hostile, disturbed, or uncomprehending, drug education may just as well not be taught.

If the school does exist to teach, what it teaches in drug education will be in the service of parental and community values. For the most part, parents want morality presented in the guise of science and "facts," in order to lend support to their own efforts at home to raise their children to be good citizens. Parents unnecessarily feel insecure and inadequate about the guidance they give to their children about drugs. Children do listen. Most children want to be what their parents want them to be; most will turn out that way. Drug education in school is more important to parents than it need be, and it is certainly of more concern to parents than it is to students. Children see the intent of drug education as being that which their parents want it to be: the teaching of why not to use drugs. Whatever the actual content of drug education—and much of it is what parents do want because teachers pursue the same ends—the simple message that children hear is: "Don't use drugs." That message is most effective at elementary school levels where moral training is based on commands and where drug use habits have not yet been established. At the high school level drug education is too late. Youngsters there are well along on their life style choices, of which drug use is but one expression.

Elementary school children bring to drug education a set of dispositions formed at home. They also bring their intellects, personalities, and motivations. For the ordinary, conforming youngsters, drug education is part of being socialized. Whether they appreciate its content will depend on their pleasures with school in general. As to the kind of course content, value clarification and decision making seems to be the poorer choice for they ask more of student and teacher than either is equipped to give.

13

Final Comment and Recommendations

In this chapter we review what has been learned and make recommendations for the school's role vis-à-vis children's drug use.

We have discovered a paradox, for drug education as we practiced it is simultaneously productive, nonproductive, and counterproductive. Furthermore, the several educational modes are both different and not so different: different if one measures impact on drug use empirically, not so different if one relies on students' reports of what they have experienced and how it has influenced them.

Drug education is productive insofar as its goal is to retard the increase in intensity and variety of nonmedical psychoactive drug use which occurs as part of the normal social development of metropolitan children. It restricts the extreme spread of use among those youngsters whose drug use is expanding anyway. That impact is limited among our California youngsters to elementary school pupils. Successful drug education is associated both with information giving and with discussion (value clarification, decision making) in the classroom, but more strikingly with the former.

Drug education is nonproductive. It makes no noticeable impact on young children in grades 2 and 3 or among older ones in grades 9-12.

And drug education is counterproductive. It destabilizes existing drug habits, including abstinence, and leads to a greater variety and intensity of use. This effect is also centered in the elementary grades, being most evident among youngsters in grades 6-8. These are the same years when the first great leap forward occurs in drug use.

Whatever is transpiring in the lives of our California drug-precocious youngsters during these years, it is a time for new personal experiences and learning. A vanguard group is responsive to drug availability and learns how to begin use. Some are sensitive to classroom information, being stimulated there to expand their drug experience. Some apparently learn moderation as well, so that they do not try out compounds popularly considered most dangerous and least socially acceptable.

Overview

Individual Differences

It is tempting to oversimplify children's drug use when in fact there are many different patterns of use, each of which will be associated with its own particular set of origins and correlates. Several patterns may also have features in common. Although our statistical measures serve to demonstrate that these correlates of drug use patterns include family characteristics, individual social conduct, and school attendance and performance, both the statistics and clinical observations warn us that a variety of unmeasured individual differences must be present. Thus, while among the most extreme drug users there is evidence for more conduct disorder, school attendance and scholastic problems, greater parental drug use, family discord on important child rearing matters, and the like, we must also find in that same extreme group children who are totally indistinguishable by our measures from children with more moderate drug-using patterns.

It is easy to go wrong in drug education. Observations in the home and classroom point to the pitfalls of statistics and education, both of which tend to rely on averages. Drug education aimed at the middle grounders easily passes by those children who are truant, those who do not comprehend, and those whose family values and habits are antagonistic to the discipline of learning or are morally at odds with the schools' conventional standards. Insofar as school personnel are themselves caught up with activities other than teaching facts, skills, or deportment, then there may be little drug education as such. When, for instance, the larger community thrusts other purposes upon the schools, leading to internal disorder—as we have seen in schools with tense racial situations or those populated with delinquent or educationally apathetic youngsters—ordinary teaching falters. It can also falter if the staff itself becomes caught up with fanciful pedagogical ideologies that are dysfunctional.

One goes wrong if it is forgotten that "prevention" cannot come after the fact. Once children have widespread drug experience, they do not value or respond behaviorally to classroom efforts. Indeed, as other research has shown, the greater that experience, the more likely that youngsters will rely on unconventional sources for their further guidance in drug affairs. The facilitating influences, the youngsters tell us, are their own pleasures in drug effects and the support and opportunities their peers provide. As one further considers how education can miss its mark, there is the reminder that what we thought we were doing and saying in the classroom seems not to have been what the students perceived. Thus, for all our efforts in teaching to encourage discussion and reflection in process education and to give information in didactic education, most of the children in the former described their experiences in terms of the latter. In addition, what we intended as minimal exposure—the control mode—was nevertheless described by its recipients in terms of information content and influence in the same way that students in more intensive courses described what they experienced.

As we consider the uniformity of the educational mode—one teacher in one classroom engaged in following one drug curriculum—we cannot help but keep in mind the contrasting multiplicity of individuals and subgroups toward which that singular effort is aimed. In examining features that distinguish children in various grades, drug levels, and drug patterns, the constellations kept changing; for example, a variable which discriminated in one cohort between high and low drug use levels did not discriminate stable from extreme spread groups. The population of drug-using children is heterogeneous. Because that is the case, there will be differences in the impact of education depending upon what the student, the drugs, the setting, and the education are like.

Community Differences

The contrast between our findings and those of Berberian and Thompson (1974) is an example of community differences. In general, their conclusions were like ours, that drug education had both retarding and enhancing impact on the normal rise in drug use. Impact in their Connecticut schools varied with kind of education, kind of drug, and grade level. They found a positive effect on children in grades 8, 9, and 10 and a drug use enhancing effect on children in grade 7. It may be that their impact on older students, one not found by us, is attributable to the differing prevalence of use in the two populations. For example, about 3 percent of the Connecticut 7th graders reported current cannabis use, whereas about 13 percent of ours reported new use (which is our closest estimate of current use). By the 10th grade, 21 percent of their population reported current cannabis use, compared with our 35 percent estimated to be currently using. Our population closest to that figure are 7th and 8th graders. The Connecticut high schoolers resemble our older elementary students, the group upon which we did have an impact. Unlike Connecticut students, the facilitating effect of our intervention was not limited to one grade level only and was different from the grades where a restraining impact was present. Perhaps the differences in educational methods account for the differences in results, but it is also possible that community drug exposure and peer stimulation were more acutely felt by the Connecticut 7th graders, while being more generally distributed among Californians from the 4th through 9th grades. In any event, drug levels and educational impact both vary with local conditions.

Curriculum Differences

The *X, Y,* and *Z* educational modes had different impacts upon drug use. That the least effort, the *X* controls, yields the least result in stimulating or controlling levels of use, indicates that teacher time and effort are directly related to children's responsiveness. On the other hand, the fact that the less-frequent method, *Y* (objective presentation of facts) had more impact than did the more-frequent *Z* (discussion and value clarification) indicates that curriculum design and content are also important. Behind the two modes are different concepts of the nature of children's social learning. The didactic mode presumes that children are rational; they receive and process information, acting upon it to guide their conduct so as to avoid what are widely believed to be high-risk drugs. Evidence for this begins with the trend in the 4th grade cohort for positive results using the Y method and becomes apparent in grades 6-8. The same didactic mode produces stimulation of interest and subsequent exploration, which is what one ordinarily wants the outcome of teaching to be. The stimulation results in youngsters more quickly becoming like older children and adults in their drug habits. Thus, normal social learning of convention, reduced fear, a spur to self-indulgence in pleasure, and curiosity may all have been transmitted along with drug facts.

The weaker showing for process education, Z, raises questions. The rationale for that approach is that children should be helped to identify their beliefs governing health and moral and social conduct, actively encouraged to incorporate some of these, and assisted in acting upon them logically. Implicit is the notion that groups in which these considerations are aired will set norms which will constitute informal peer standards. Also implicit is the expectation that what the child will decide is what the community wants him to decide; choices will be in the direction of conventional wisdom. If the teacher is more psychodynamically inclined and/or nondirective, the alternative assumption may be that discussion does not guide the child to particular risk-avoiding and moral conduct, but simply to greater maturity and thoughtful independence. If the teacher is optimistic about the marriage between conventionality and wisdom, it may be hoped that such informed self-reliance will, nevertheless, lead to "normal" drug use. Most of the decision making formats find the teacher acting much like modern parents when they respectfully invite egalitarian participation by the child in formulating his own beliefs and setting his action goals. Whether this method is one of manipulative hypocrisy or genuine confidence in the maturity of all concerned depends upon the people involved.

Why, of the two approaches, does the simpler, cheaper, less "helpful" and less "dynamic" mode work better? It is a surprise, especially since so many experts have denounced informational approaches to drug education in favor of more complex models. We are not sure, but on the basis of clinical observations, our own and those of Zinberg *et al.* (1976), it is clear that children are quite uneasy talking in the classroom about anything personally consequential. They are shy and defensive, want to present themselves to their peers in the best possible light, and act to protect themselves from peer ridicule and cruelty, teacher censure, or parental disapproval. Shame is to be avoided, and so are revelations and betrayal.

The school's contract with children does not ordinarily offer the special features of personal expression or character development in return for "openness." Child and teacher carry to their discussions a prior understanding of what school is really about: structure, obedience, learning, or, in the absence of these, disrespect, delinquency, chaos. Not reflective self-expression, not character development, not therapy. There is license of a sort. Private suffering is allowed, and so is escape (e.g., illness, truancy, apathy, and mischief). The tyranny of peers exists in the schoolyard, but inside school the ruling elders' civic virtue strives to be pervasive.

Such forces and reactions do not illumine the private core of self or coax the child to surrender his inner decisions immediately to others, as superficial value clarification lures him to do. Ultimately, most children do conform; the normal curve of drug use is proof of this. But the inner self remains unspeaking, unspoken to, treasuring its fortress-like silence. Those for whom the forces of conformity do not prove irresistible—and are indistinguishable from either social learning or maturation—become, in the drug arena, outlaws. The correlational statistics on extreme drug use, deviancy, and delinquency testify to that. These "deviants" are usually insufficiently complex, their inner selves are weak and not private enough, so that they publicly act out either neurosis or the characterological lack of having been civilized. That acting out is careless and too loud, being the essence of damaging indiscretion. Few are the poets for whom nonconformity in childhood has meant artistic strength.

Under these circumstances, teachers are probably at their best doing what they are ordinarily trained to do: offering information, supervising the class, and being a moral model. The child sees himself as safest when responding in kind; thus, Z follows Y in the alphabet of our impact findings. Our survey of student reactions confirmed their adherence to the "rational" model for education. This finding as to what is routine does not prove that what is routine is also ideal.

Our data are no refutation of the advocates of child-centered education who want the school as milieu to be altered. We do not at all address the effectiveness of programs which identify and seek to refer and help the child who has actual troubles in association with drug use, these very likely symptomatic of problems in living. Our limited data do indicate that teachers may well be able to identify those children with serious problems in living and, by correlation with actual or potential drug use extremes, but in the absence of special programs to encourage case finding and referral, there is little chance that the school will initiate special help.

Timing

Timing for drug education intervention is a critical aspect relating to effectiveness. The consistent trend for both stimulation to popular drug use and restraint from the use of unusual substances is keyed to age. There was a consistent trend for the success of Y over Z over X for grades 4-8, with the greatest in the 6th grade (grades 6-8) cohort. Radically different reactions to drug education on the part of the student consumers were also keyed to grade, their approval and recommendations being remarkably closely linked to actual impact.

This age for impact was also the age of instability, that is, when students in large numbers were first beginning to change their drug use habits, moving from abstinence or low-level sanctioned use to higher and less-approved use. One cannot show a preventive effect unless one does make a measure during a period when a change is about to occur; on the other hand, the ever-widening experience of the older youngsters was not retarded, whereas the 6th grade cohort's stirrings were affected, both in a stimulating and a controlling fashion.

Prevention, as we tested it, requires an intervention before the fact, yet also at an age when other features—the determining forces in society, neighborhood, peers, family, and person—have generated a readiness to embark on a new kind of behavior. With drugs this behavior is social, for drugs are acquired from and used in the company of other youngsters. It is also individual; the novice user does something and experiences an effect which is rewarding. The effect may or may not be solely pharmacological; chances are that there are both biochemically induced and psychological pleasures, e.g., peer approval, acting out of fantasies of being independent and grown up, and the like. The new behavior is very much in the moral sphere; the child taking drugs on his own knows he is being daring, pleasure indulging, and "bad." One is struck by the paradox that the "immoral" rebellion against family, school, and community prohibitions leads quickly, for most, to a return to morality, that is, to conventional behavior defined as doing what adults and older children do. The eleven-year-old metropolitan area California child disobeys the rules laid down for children in order to develop and accede to the drug use habits of Californians of high school age and above. The eleven-year-old mimics the delinquencies of older children and the customs of adults. The drug behavior can be one and the same.

The maximal impact of education, as we have shown it, is simply to further speed and possibly to confirm or stabilize rapid development into alcohol, tobacco, and marijuana use, but to facilitate as well the rejection of those extremes of drug use which characterize only the unusual older children and adults. We cannot, of course, say how long lasting any of that educational effect may be, but during the period of our observation its effect is to do very much what normal schooling does: to move children toward adulthood by giving them facts and skills which characterize or are useful to adults.

Rational and Responsible?

How this effect is achieved in the format of information giving, more so than via discussion, is an open question. We do not think it is simply an artifact of time, place, or experimental error. Perhaps, if Zinberg *et al.*'s idea of inevitable information distortion upon reception is correct, there are more data to be misperceived, thus speeding the age of irrationality so that children sooner become as foolish as adults in relying heavily on psychoactive drugs for recreation and relief. If one thinks those adult habits wise, then one may argue that age eleven or so is a time when children are ready to hear and act on factual communications that propel them to the sagacious self-indulgence of their chemically preoccupied—if not confused—elders. Alternatively, one might believe that eleven is an age when California youngsters are ready, when effectively stimulated by their teachers, to dramatically express that striving for status and full equality so characteristic of egalitarian and role-merging modern America. Whether to mimic adulthood via drug use around age eleven is in fact a benefit remains a question. Those who argue that children must stay innocent and protected buck a libertarian trend; those who argue children's right to stoned equality might well consider what the age of legal responsibility has become.

There confront us, then, four important and continuing questions which relate to timing and responsibility. One depends on social and epidemiological data and asks, What is the time when drugs become available to children in a community and the first significant movement into regular self-administration begins? The second asks if and when educational intervention can best be timed to intrude preventively upon or intercept this critical period, in a given school, of drug habit instability. The third asks about the appropriate age, given current knowledge of child development and psychopharmacology, for shifts from child to adult status to be either encouraged or resisted in those moral-social-health matters bearing on the pursuit of experience through chemistry. The fourth question asks about the age at which a doctrine of legal and fiscal responsibility can appropriately be invoked in response to damage, costs, or "vice" associated with early drug use. The answers to the first two questions depend on research, the answer to the third upon research and community standards. The fourth reply rests on developments in moral and legal thought, including thoughts about what is the etiology and meaning of drug use.

Strategy: Policy Options for School Intervention

We turn now to a consideration of policy. Given what is known about children's drug use, the effects of school intervention, and the politics of the real world, what should a school district, individual schools, and responsible teachers and administrators do?

Getting One's Ideology Straight

The first step is to reflect upon one's own and one's community's basic views as to what children's drug use represents, from what it arises, what correctives are in order, and what the proper role of the school is. If those views are dictated by extreme political ideologies rather than by existing scientific findings, such that there is neither room for choice in what schools do, nor interest in empirical data, then there are no policy options. Let us illustrate two extremes of that sort.

In one case, a vocal political group is convinced that children's drug use, whatever form it takes, arises because an exploiting capitalist society encourages pharmaceutical manufacturers to sell addictive poisons (all drugs are so defined) in order to make profits. Simultaneously, the intent is to lull citizens into chemical stupor or false euphoria so that they cannot resist their oppressors, the U.S. Government. "Uncle Sam, the pusher man" is the symbol of this exploitative mental castration. This belief leads to the following action program: (1) transform the schools into a base for revolutionary action via political propagandizing, and convince the students they are an exploited minority who must renounce drug use and seize power; and (2) destroy existing institutions, including schools as they are now constituted, and replace them with radical structures run by the "people," who will enforce the new system militantly. Illicit drug activities become subject to severe and consistent punitive sanctions, including the death penalty. Ridiculous? Perhaps, but this extreme case is openly espoused and pursued as the theme in one California school system. The means advocated for altering drug behavior include political-personal counseling, separation of children from parents when the latter hold reactionary views and the provision of live-in centers for those children, group criticism sessions, terrorism, and violent revolution.

The second extreme case is that which powers a Texas town's drug education. Their materials imply that humans are gullible and weak, easily controlled by chemicals. These are purposely pushed by conspirators who intend to enslave the young through "addiction" (almost all drug use is so defined) and, in that way, to undermine the nation; it would then fall prey to communists, the Mafia, or other "menacing" plotters. The action program derived calls for (1) increased police surveillance, including campus agents, to identify conspiring drug dealers; (2) involvement of school authorities in the search for "extremists"; (3) advocacy of total abstinence from drugs (excluding tobacco and alcohol) combined with very punitive laws constitutionally enforced by unrestrained narcotics police; and (4) involvement of the church in a (probably unconstitutional) liaison with schools for a moral crusade.

Both of these cases reveal the apparatus of tyranny, left and right, mobilized around the "cause" of children's drug use control. In contrast, the policy options here considered exclude such politically derived programs in favor of what we hope are gentler doctrines resting on empiricism, cost-benefit analysis, flexibility, a basic optimism about children's healthy development and the benevolent intentions of most school personnel, and a mild pessimism about institutional as opposed to one-to-one personal intervention in lives. Ours is also the conviction that children's drug use is a complex matter of morals and social learning, a health hazard, a statutory delinquency, and an expression of the biological propensity for humans to explore and employ chemicals which affect the brain.

Listing the Alternatives

Let us review what has been proposed for and/or done within American schools in response to drug use. Table 13-1 lists in column one major preventive or responsive programs either tried or proposed. Column 2 summarizes such results as have been reported for these activities or can be estimated. Column 3 suggests the objectives and community circumstances which support or justify each kind of activity. It will be seen that the activities are scaled from none (*A*) to maximum (*E*) in terms of effort and innovation required. The table is abbreviated and, when there is absence of rational evidence, presents our best guesses.

The Reserved Posture: Selecting an Appropriate Strategy

At level *A* in the table, when there is no intervention either preventively or in response to specific problems, that may be due to the school's or community's caution or conviction. The conviction is usually one of policy: that moral education in the drug sphere is not school business. Although that moral issue is not always acknowledged as such, for educational discussions about drugs are often packaged as health or scientific concerns, adult concern about drug use certainly does center on opinions about what is right and wrong for children. Safety is also a consideration, so is lawfulness, and so is the symbolic meaning of drug use as independence, rebellion, self-indulgence, or whatever. Nevertheless, the decision not to engage in drug education, when based on conviction, expresses a position on the role of schools in moral training. The position itself may be conservative or "progressive," the conservative posture holding that children must be given moral training, but that it is the domain of family and church. The progressive posture is that the school should not care about children's drug use, for that is a sphere of private conduct which is not public business. In either case, there is no strategy for the educator to choose or for us to recommend, for the school is being responsive to strongly held community values or, in the case of private institutions, to the beliefs of client parents.

When, on the other hand, the decision not to engage in drug education is based on caution, as responsive to fiscal, drug use, and educational impact data, there are strategy options to consider. Ordinarily, the cautious decision will have been made when authorities are aware that levels of drug use and change in the

Table 13-1
Drug Education Strategies

School activities	"Best guess" as to outcome (assuming a "best effort.")	Necessary (a) Objectives, and (b) Community circumstances
A. None: no drug education and no special programs.	Avoids stimulating children's interest in and use of popular drugs. Deprives troubled children of referral/treatment opportunities.	a) To avoid costs or stimulation of adult style drug use. Belief that moral education is not a school function. b) Community drug use levels low, and community drug problems few, and community drug treatment resources inadequate.
B. Targeted and ancillary—real problem intervention only.		
1) Training teachers to identify and refer problem children. Training school counselors to assist these children using the referral process.	1) Increased use of referral opportunities.	1a) To limit in-school programs to after-the-fact assistance to problem children.
2) Establishing school-community programs to refer troubled children to helping agencies or after-school therapeutic and alternative activities.	2) Decrease in adjustment and school problems among treated youngsters.	2a) To assure help for those children, be that for health, learning, behavior or other difficulties.
3) Assisting interested parents by offering (a) education in parenting or assisting, and (b) referral of children with drug problems.	3) (a) show improvement in child-rearing methods and parent confidence, and (b) some increase in referral with subsequent child adjustment improvement.	3a) To avoid stimulating drug use in general. 4a) To target efforts so as to minimize school costs.
4) School support for community programs for alternatives to drug use, e.g., recreation, sports, music, meditation, farming, hobbies, supervised peer clubs.	4) Long-range improvement in the quality of lives.	5a) Commitment to general community improvement. 6a) Commitment to working closely with other community agencies and with parents.
5) School support for community efforts directed at the child with problems in living who is at high drug risk, e.g., drop-in centers, police arrest and diversion, "hot line" switchboards, family counseling, neighborhood improvement, job opportunity improvements and	5) Constructive resolution of individual and family crises, possible long-range improvement in the quality of community services.	b) Existence of adequate community resources for treatment and drug alternative activities. Awareness of existence of troubled children with drug-associated problems and other problems in living. No rapid expansion of children's use of high-risk substances as evidenced by continuing community surveys.

teenage vocational counseling/placement, improved community mental health facilities, improved police juvenile bureaus. May include special schools or living-in facilities for troubled youngsters or those removed from unwholesome homes.

C. School-wide changes which are neither radical nor drug specific.

1) Teacher training to improve teachers' communication, social skills, drug information, self-awareness in drug areas, empathy with children, liaison with parents.

2) Training for and consultation with school administrators and school boards to insure support for general school programs fostering schools as child centered; e.g., elaboration of drug alternative courses and after-school activities in music, sports-for-all, hobbies, meditation. Also, support for school counseling services and for supervision of excellence of case finding and referral for troubled children. Also increased "outreach" programs for parents and students to participate as consumers in program evaluation, provision of special mental health consultation to teachers to assist them in handling problem children, etc.

3) Control of delinquency on the schoolgrounds and of disorder in the classroom.

1) Some improvement in teacher styles, greater improvement in specific knowledge.

2a) Increased opportunities for staff, students, and parents to expand their interests and range of conscious choice.

2b) Risk of reduction of emphasis on educational "fundamentals" and lip service to improvements generating costs without real change.

3) Provision of an environment in which learning and social decency are possible. Provision of external controls necessary for the development, in predelinquent and other children, of internal controls. Teaching, by example, that misbehavior is both wrong and unrewarding.

1-2a) Willingness to involve teachers and administrators in serious continuing education, oriented to their beliefs and behavior *without* compromising their autonomy or commitment to teaching fundamentals.

1-2b) No intensive demand by the community for direct intervention with drugs per se. Community understanding that drug problems are associated with other problems in living. Willingness to experiment with the school milieu in the hopes that improved social/psychological atmospheres will enhance child development and learning.

3a) To maintain schools as places where civilization is seen and experienced as well as talked about. Commitment to immediate delinquency and drug use control.

3b) Support by the community for efforts to make the schools models for lawful and decent interpersonal conduct. This implies police, parental, and judicial sanctions to back up school authorities.

Table 13-1 (cont.)

School activities	"Best guess" as to outcome (assuming a "best effort.")	Necessary (a) Objectives, and (b) Community circumstances
4) Special course and classwork designed to facilitate moral and character development. (School milieu must be compatible.)	4) Probable increase in level of moral development (on psychological tests). Possible control of delinquency. Character growth effects untested.	4a) Conviction that morals and character are proper concern of schools. 4b) Sufficient community homogeneity and confidence to allow schools to exercise moral authority (necessarily along conventional lines) and to experiment with character education in selected class activities.
D. Drug-specific activities aimed at all children: 1) Training teachers as drug educators, either for didactic, value clarification, or group dynamic methods.	1) Some increase in teacher knowledge, confidence, skill, and self-awareness.	1a) Commitment to teacher improvement.
2) Short-term drug education: didactic.	2) Some increase in children's drug interests and activities. Knowledge increase.	2-3a) Interest in showing an effort without concern for effects.
3) Short-term drug education: value clarification and attitude change modes.	3) Some increase in children's drug interests and activities. Some attitude changes occur: greater acceptance of drugs and users.	
4) Long-term drug education: psychoanalytic group dynamic mode.	4) Increase in exploratory drug use, in self-reflection. Possible long-term increase in self-confidence, range of choice, and self-control.	4a) Interest in personal development along mental health lines. No specific objective regarding drug use.
5) Long-term drug education: didactic model using selected health, psychology or, science text books which are objective.	5) Probable increase in knowledge and stimulation of popular drug use. Hopefully rational control over high-risk behavior.	5a) Interest in incorporating actual drug education into existing health or science education.
6) Long-term drug education: Stanford value clarification curriculum, grade-timed intervention.	6) Some increase in use of popular drugs and some control by otherwise extreme drug users in the use of unpopular (high-risk) substances. Felt increase in knowledge and approval of course content and teachers. Felt influence on drug-taking decisions.	6a) Interest in preventive intervention with conviction that discussion method's superiority outweighs its lesser actual impact on use during the educational intervention period. Special interest in those person-oriented students who respond best to discussion methods.

7) Long-term drug education: didactic mode, Stanford curriculum, and grade-timed intervention.

E. Radical school reform in which drug education is a correlated, minor, or red herring issue.
   1) Remodeling the public school so that it becomes the "good family." Educational objectives are secondary until character and morality are assured.
   2) Remodeling the public school to conform to political, religious, or psychological ideologies (i.e., Marxist theories that drug abuse disappears with the elimination of capitalism; reactionary views that drug abuse arises only because leftists sell drugs to undermine the weak, progressive theories; linked to humanistic mental health notions that development of individual potentials negates any self-damaging or socially undesirable conduct).
   3) Eliminating present mandatory and specific school attendance in favor of some free-choice system, e.g., vouchers usable among competing approved public and private systems, or extending voucher use to unlicensed individuals and centers as well. Alternatively, assured

7) Increase in use of popular drugs during intervention period. Reduced use of less-popular (high-risk) drugs among otherwise extreme users. Felt increase in knowledge and approval of teachers and course content. Felt influence on drug-taking decisions.

1-2) Empirical studies are lacking. The success of "brainwashing" and "total institutions" in totalitarian countries indicates that one can replace the family and mold personalities. The graduates of existing parochial, private, and special schools also reflect the success of ideologically committed educational programs.

3) ?????

7a) Interest in preventive intervention, willingness to accept facilitation of older age drug use styles as trade off for control of unpopular (higher-risk) drugs.

1-7b) Facilities and commitment in community to regular monitoring of children's drug use trends. Willingness to intervene preventively—knowing that this will stimulate older age-use styles—when trends indicate availability of hallucinogens, opiates, stimulants, sedatives, and high risk of children using these nonmedically.

1-2a) Willingness to subordinate present educational (skill, intellectual) objectives to moral, social, political, and psychological ideals.

1-2b) Either dominant political power or public concurrence in support. Note this may be present in any subgroup which controls its own schools regionally or parochially. Private schools can also serve this function.

3a) Desire radically to alter the status quo and a conviction that peer, parental, and/or student choice would be beneficial. Optimism about temporary anarchy. Optimism about the economics of competition among schools. Opti-

Table 13-1 (cont.)

School activities	"Best guess" as to outcome (assuming a "best effort.")	Necessary (a) Objectives, and (b) Community circumstances
public support to all regardless of age, vocational, or educational status plus tuition for those wishing to attend approved (and publically supported) training or educational agencies representing a broad spectrum of interests, skills, and knowledge.		mism about the ability to provide public fiscal support to persons not fitting themselves for employment. 3b) A different philosophy than that which is current.

school population are low, and, further, when parental anxiety about drug use and ability to control it in their children is also low. The noninvolvement decision will also rest on substantial knowledge demonstrating that there are few child health or conduct difficulties connected with drug use. There is also awareness that drug education can—as the research shows—stimulate use in a direction that most parents probably do not want, i.e., hurrying the child into older drug use patterns. There will also be awareness that any drug program, be it teaching or case finding, will involve the effort of change and some costs. It is not fiscally prudent to incur effort or costs to engage in activities which are not needed and which, in the teaching instance, may be counterproductive.

Under the foregoing conditions, we concur in the strategy of school inaction, recommending that no effort be made as long as the drug use and outcome situation remain both benign and stable. The qualification "stable" implies that such a strategy must be flexible, for in the face of new situations it may be well to revise the policy. Given the fact that drug use in the United States is expanding downward by age, outward by region, across classes, and toward new drugs, it is likely that there will come a time, at least for most nonsectarian schools, that the same caution that dictated program abstemiousness will then dictate intervention. To know if and when policy changes are in order, the school must have access to data on trends in youthful drug use, on frequency and kind of hazardous health-accident outcomes in association with drug use, and on the drug use of delinquent and academically impoverished youngsters.

Monitoring Trends

Implicit in the foregoing is a must: schools and communities must commission studies and monitor drug use trends, health and accident histories, and delinquents' and poor academic performers' drug histories. Quite likely, when rate and problem increases arise parental anxiety will also increase, for, as we have shown, one of the strong correlates of extreme drug use is mothers' awareness of children's drug interests and use. These parental worries should also be matters of interest to the school. As the general rate of use of high-risk substances increases, one expects initially higher rates of use in the delinquent and academically marginal youngsters, as well as in the children of wealthier, liberal families. For the former group already in trouble, their drug use will be symptomatic, but that group will also be at special risk of acute or long-range damage or dysfunction in association with drugs, alcohol and tobacco of course included.

When there are signs of increases in use, accidents, delinquent drug involvement, etc., the rule of prudence will be for preventive and responsive programs to be considered. These can be specific for schools and, indeed, for subgroups within schools. At first, considerable differences are to be expected among children in various neighborhoods differentiated by income, religion, and ethnicity. As fashions and practices spread across these social trait boundaries, differences may blur and city-wide programs will be in order.

The Minimal Acceptable Response When Problems Exist

When there is indication that use and problem levels are rising, and perhaps parental concerns as well, the school will want to exercise one or more of the options ranging from B through D in Table 13-1. The school may select any one or all of the activities listed in B and C activity levels, for each is compatible with the others. It is likely that the number and level of activities selected for action will depend upon the speed and extent to which drug use changes are occurring within a student body and spreading through a town. Decisions will also be affected by the resources in a community, including facilities, funds, and personnel, as well as by the speed with which public interest and political groups facilitate innovation in schools and out.

When drug use levels in a school population are rising slowly, but there is evidence that the high-risk group of delinquents and academic marginals are beginning to use intensively (as exemplified by accident and clinic records, probation department interview reports, and the like), the minimal justifiable response of the school will be to initiate community liaison and to begin training teachers and counselors for case finding and referral. Those youngsters who are observed to suffer acute drug effects should have the opportunity for treatment. The school must have a channel which takes advantage of the demonstrated teacher sensitivity to student problems and move at-risk youngsters into counseling and community programs.

Case Finding and Referrals

At the very least, that program will include teacher training for alertness to possible acute drug effects (behavioral signs such as depression, hyperactivity, sleeping, confusion, hallucinations, erratic violence, and inappropriateness, and medical signs such as slurred speech, convulsions, injection-induced infection, stupor, etc.) and to the nature of referral channels, parental liaison, and community drug, family, and mental health consultation services. There needs to be a monitored program to encourage teacher referrals to a school coordinator such as the nurse, counselor, psychologist, drug specialist, or, in the absence of such gatekeepers, to a designated administrator. At the very least, the program will insure that the designated referral coordinator in the school will have established community and parental liaison. Ideally, that person will have sufficient sophistication in counseling and history taking to understand how the child's drug use fits into his life style and which agencies are best tailored to that child's situation (detoxification centers, mental health and family service agencies, police juvenile officers, pastoral counseling, drug treatment centers, etc.). The within-school coordinator will be able to initiate discussions with the parents and, when the family is irresponsible or otherwise unresponsive, there will need to be direct channels to community counseling, medical, and legal authorities for assistance with the family difficulty. It will be important for coordinators and others to keep in mind that destructive drug use occurs in the context of other problems and that while the drug or drug outcome may be the immediate focus, the long-range focus will very likely be on personality, family, or social factors.

Delinquency Control

Delinquency control on the schoolgrounds is the second aspect of that minimal response program which is attentive to acute health, behavior, and school performance problems. Because it is likely to be more difficult, this is listed as a level *C* endeavor in Table 13-1. The school should not knowingly allow possession or distribution of any prohibited psychoactive drug on school-grounds. That means, for most states, that persons under sixteen should be discouraged from smoking anywhere, contrary to an expanding practice whereby schools provide sanctuaries for this unhealthy and illicit drug correlated conduct. (Forty-seven of the fifty states prohibit sale of cigarettes to persons below a specified age, ranging from fifteen to twenty-one.) Minors will not be allowed liquor or to be drunk on schoolgrounds. No student is to be allowed possession in school of cannabis or other nonprescribed psychoactives.

The problems of delinquency control in schools generally—vandalism, arson, violence, theft, rape, and extortion—have become so great for many schools that there has been a tendency to disregard the quieter, private activities of drug use. Although such disregard is understandable in terms of policing difficulties, the increasing advocacy for the repeal of criminal laws governing nonvictim crimes, a desire to accommodate to what may seem inevitable, and opposition to the *in locus parentes* authority of schools, nevertheless the school's failure to exert control can signal approval in practice for those drug use traits which most parents and teachers condemn verbally. There is no wisdom in an inconsistency which serves to teach a practical lesson in hypocricy and nonrestraint. A policy of drug delinquency control does not mean that school authorities call the police when an offense becomes known; such a punishment is worse than the crime. But delinquency control does mean that a clear policy is communicated to all students. The policy might be that any first violation is cited by school authorities with a warning to desist, a second violation is communicated to parents, and a third to a teacher-peer review committee which may impose penalties.

Drug delinquency control should include student peer participation whenever possible. Such groups, democratically selected and specially trained for their leadership role, participate in setting norms and reviewing offenses as well as in determining the action to take with offenders. Simple penalties may be in order, depending on the range of school authority, as, for example, cleaning schoolgrounds, washing school vehicles, or being denied privileges. Often cases will be referred to counselors, special group programs, or sometimes to juvenile authorities.

The effect of a control policy may be to encourage discretion; that is, to make drug delinquencies invisible rather than blatant. This is all our society requires for many otherwise disapproved actions. School authorities can, if that happens to be their opinion, acknowledge that private behavior ought not to be the law's business. Nevertheless, drug use will remain public business as long as the actions or reactions are themselves public. Insofar as youngsters persist in indiscretions and invite attention, they are likely to be revealing those common correlates of drug delinquency such as rebellion, risk taking, impulsiveness, or emotional disorder. The repeat offender will be advertising himself dramatically enough to give school personnel and peers an opportunity to ask about the reasons why. Such persistent expressions require that the family, professionals, and community agencies respond. These efforts do not need justification on righteous grounds. It is sufficient that the youngster be flagrant in his delinquency and unresponsive to ordinary social controls, to justify school concern. Keep in mind that it is the youngster who needs attending to, not simply the drugs he uses.

There are circumstances in which drug delinquency control cannot be exercised because the school cannot defend its children, its personnel, or its physical plant from predatory and violent crime. One can be sure that in such circumstances the correlation between the other delinquency and high-risk drug use, including alcohol, will be great. That knowledge is irrelevant if there is no way to prevent schoolground delinquency as such. Unfortunately, we have no suggestion to make here. We acknowledge that the school cannot function as a place of learning when it is a jungle. Delinquency control under those circumstances becomes the first priority to insure the survival of learning as well as of civilization.

A school may decide, either because of parental concern, rising use, and problem levels, or because opportunities for constructive change are at hand, to move beyond the minimal levels of problem response and control to simultaneously preventive and constructive endeavors, as, for example, some of the components of level B in Table 13-1 and items 1, 2, and 4 at level C. These efforts, broad and innovative, avoid any direct intervention in class which risks stimulating drug use. These general efforts, like the minimal acceptable response, are suitable for school populations where some problems exist or are anticipated, but where levels of use are not yet so great that one wants to chance increasing them via educational stimulation. These programs are advantageous in schools and communities where the majority of children will not, by the time they finish high school, become regular users of illicit substances or intensive users of alcohol and tobacco. The advantage of these B and C level activities is that they are also generally constructive, providing enrichment for children's lives within and outside the school.

At The Crisis Point—Drug Education In The Classroom

When monitoring yields the information that drug use levels are rapidly expanding so that the prediction is that before the end of high school the majority of youngsters will be regular users of alcohol, tobacco, and marijuana, with a substantial minority employing the pills, powders, and injectables, then this can be the time for drug education in the classroom. This decision depends upon the mood of parents; if they are worried and if they want the school to provide that backup to their own efforts which only school-wide classroom activities do, then there is added reason to inaugurate drug teaching. The decision also depends upon the success and feasibility of alternative, nonspecific activities at B and C levels in Table 13-1. If the school prefers to undertake or can show the success of these general efforts to enrich the lives of children without the risk of drug use stimulation, it will not go on to level D activities. On the other hand general efforts, because they are not targeted, are likely to yield less control of extreme drug use expansion over the short term. That is our estimate; no data bear on it. Finally, the decision rests upon the willingness of the school to train its teachers as competent drug educators and to provide them with sound teaching materials and sufficient time for presentation. In the Stanford didactic program that is once a month.

If the conditions for preventive classroom intervention are met, the strategic option which is recommended is to engage in level D activities as shown in Table 13-1. Unlike the alternatives at B and C levels, several of those under D are logically incompatible one with the other. On the basis of our own work and that of others, it is our recommendation that the school committed to classroom drug education opt for items 1 (training teachers) and either 5 or 7. Item 7 is the long-term didactic mode using the Stanford curriculum timed for application to precede and accompany the early expansion in drug use.

In our schools this burst occurred at about ages eleven to thirteen; in other communities, it can be earlier or later. This is shown on the curves of Figure 6-1a and Figures 8-1 and 8-2.[a] It is this explosion, whereby the majority begins to use

[a]Alcohol experience prevalence rises from 19 percent to 63 percent, cigarettes from 17 percent to 50 percent, inhalants from 27 percent to 45 percent (or higher); regular marijuana use makes its first appearance and experimentation moves from near-zero levels to 10 percent or 15 percent; the pills (amphetamines, barbiturates, hallucinogens) show their first regular use and experimentation from near zero to 10 percent or 15 percent; and opiates-cocaine make their first appearance in regular use and almost their first appearance in exploratory use.

the (adult) sanctioned substances and a minority begins regular unsanctioned drug use, which we identify as the phase at which our form of classroom drug education is optimal. Later research might well modify this picture; one might find, for example, some increased power for long-range control to be shown for enduring education that begins preventively and continues even as drug use rises.

Our data and opinions lead us to recommend against the other activities, items 2, 3, 4, and 6 at level D in Table 13-1. We would expect that other curricula may do as well as ours, so that, although comparative data are lacking, a similar type of intervention using other materials, i.e., item 5, could be considered. That intervention should be tested for effects via sound evaluation.

Broad Reform

We make no recommendations pertaining to level E. Those proposals are beyond the scope of this book and our own knowledge of how best to reform schools and society.

Implementing Strategies: Where To Begin

This chapter intends to be a general guide to what to do, but is not a how-to-do-it manual; the mechanics of some of levels B and C are complicated. Level D activities that we recommend are simple, requiring only that teachers be trained at reputable drug education training institutes and that they then follow either our own Stanford didactic curriculum or other sound texts. Whatever strategic option is selected, the first steps are those outlined earlier in this chapter: first, getting one's own thoughts on children's drug use straight by virtue of attending to the facts and reflecting on one's own ideology, and second, consulting local data on trends and outcomes to see what children really are doing and experiencing with drugs and how this is part of their lives.

At the next level, the educational policy maker will want to know what his community resources and demands are, how feasible various activities at levels B and C are, what they will cost, and who in the community can join in the effort. Liaisons will be helpful with community mental health and drug treatment centers, juvenile police and probation authorities, family service agencies, epidemiologists and survey research workers, and colleges and universities engaged in drug research programs. Since the work of the Drug Prevention Branch of the Office of Education, Washington, D.C., has been uniformly excellent, communications to that office, as well as to the National Institute on Drug Abuse (Rockwall Building, 11400 Rockville Pike, Rockville, Maryland 20852), can be relied upon to produce good information and advice. Most states by now have agencies for drug abuse control usually operating as part of the

Health and Welfare Department. They, too, can provide information and sometimes field assistance.

We recommend strongly against seeking assistance from sources with a record of consistent bias or ignorance. Usually state and local police narcotics departments fall into this unfortunate category, and so too in recent years has the Federal Drug Enforcement Administration. Police juvenile bureaus are often much more objective. Political and religious groups who exploit the drug arena for their own aggrandizement are also unreliable sources for the honest schoolteacher or administrator. Nor can one assume that professionals are well informed; physicians, for example, are often unschooled in psychopharmacology and certainly in child psychology. Clinical psychologists, psychiatrists, or social workers are trained to be sensitive to individual lives and problems but are usually unacquainted with social and epidemiological data or program evaluation methods. And beware of those who are "expert" simply because they have "experience" as drug educators. That experience may work only to confirm them in the most egregious and opinionated errors. Indeed, some of the materials we have seen in the drug education field achieve eminence only as all-time atrocities, ravaging reason, insulting science, and poisoning the trust of the child in teachers.

A Cantonese Closing: Sweet and Sour

Trends in drug use in most metropolitan areas, as well as many mid-size towns, probably justify didactic classroom education of the kind we have tested. Such offerings are, in a sense, "crisis" intervention, except that we would not encourage the notion or the language of panic in response to children's drug use. "Crisis" intervention does have a more useful connotation, one derived from community psychiatry. It is a professional effort to set people on a constructive course during a time when they are unsettled and uncertain. The "instability" period in children's drug habits, in our sample around ages eleven to thirteen, provides such an opportunity. Drug education is also an opportunity for the exercise of broader constructive child- rather than drug-centered activities, those at levels *B* and *C* in Table 13-1. These latter are the kinds of drug endeavors that have been encouraged by the U.S. Office of Education under the leadership of Helen Nowlis.

In contemplating classroom drug education, it is well to think of the short and the long term. The outlook does not justify any expectation that drug-specific education, be that in the context of health, morals, science, or consumer protection, will prevent the expanding variety and intensity of drug use which characterizes our society. Children will move into adult drug use habits whether they proceed quickly or slowly. The best we can hope for is to control that movement sufficiently so that the child's interim developmental costs are not too high. We can also hope that the child comes to practice only the particular drug use customs of those older than he which are more rather than less safe. That is a long-term goal. To accomplish that selectivity naturally requires that the child be favored in his or her family, peers, neighborhood, subculture, and personality. As we have seen, these are the powerful forces shaping drug use, ones with which the school competes successfully only during those "unstable" or "critical" years as drug use begins to expand dramatically.

There is reason to believe that the school can assist in guiding development so that some youngsters, despite speeding up their conventional acquisitions, will refrain from more extreme drug conduct. Although we do not know, in fact, whether this restraint is long lasting, an article of faith declares that it should be. Delay, restraint, and judgment once practiced become inner resources capable of further application. Since we have observed that this control arises in the course of didactic education, a mode which proclaims the rational child, there is nourishment for the belief that humans can be rational—at least some can, at least somewhat, even about drugs, and even in consequence of schooling. We do not know whether that is achieved by the content of the curriculum and matters of which we are aware, or by subtler processes which we did not observe. One is troubled here of course by the equivalence of restraint and rationality with what is really quite varied and active conventional drug use, and most of which has costs as well as benefits. Thus, the rationality described may be better conceived as acquiescence in being normal, doing what most others do. Whether one finally and in fact will equate wisdom with conformity deserves weighty, individual deliberation. In any event, insofar as drug education does facilitate that rationality which abjures high-risk drug use, we can find reason, as well as hope, in education.

References

References

Abrams, L.A., Garfield, E.F., and Swisher, J.D., Eds. *Accountability In Drug Education: A Model for Evaluation.* Washington, D.C.: Drug Abuse Council, Inc., Nov. 1973.

Abruzzi, D. and Abruzzi, W. "Middle Class Heroin Addiction: The New Epidemic." Hudson Valley, New York, 1975. (Mimeograph.)

Ahlstrom, W.M. and Havinghurst, R.S. *Four Hundred Losers.* San Francisco: Jossey-Bass, 1971.

American School Health Association and Pharmaceutical Manufacturers Association. *Teaching About Drugs: A Curriculum Guide, K-12,* Second edition. Kent, Ohio: American School Health Association, 1971.

Aubrey, R. "Drug Education: Can Teachers Really Do the Job?" *Teachers College Record* (1971-72): 417.

Becker, Howard. *Outsiders: Studies in the Sociology of Deviance.* Glencoe, Illinois: Free Press, 1963.

Bedworth, A.E. and D'Elia, J.A. "Editorial: Guidelines for Programs in Drug Education." *Journal of Drug Education* (March 1971): 1.

_____ and D'Elia, J.A. *Basics of Drug Education.* New York: Baywood Publishing Company, 1973.

Berberian, R.M. and Thompson, W.D. "The Relationship Between Drug Education and Changes in Drug Use." Paper presented at the North American Congress on Alcohol and Drug Problems, San Francisco, December 1974.

Birdwood, G. "The Don'ts of Drug Education." *Drugs and Society* (January 1972): 1.

Birk, E. *Official Report, House of Lords Debates,* Vol. 314, Columns 260-266. London: Her Majesty's Stationery Office, January 14, 1971.

Blum, E.M. "The Uncooperative Patient: The Development of a Test to Predict Uncooperativeness in Medical Treatment." *Supplementary Studies of Malpractice.* San Francisco: California Medical Association, 1958.

Blum, R.H. and Associates. *Utopiates: The Use and Users of LSD-25.* New York: Atherton, 1964.

_____ and Associates. *Students and Drugs: College and High School Observations.* San Francisco: Jossey-Bass, 1969.

_____ and Associates. *Horatio Alger's Children: Family Factors in the Origin and Prevention of Drug Risk.* San Francisco: Jossey-Bass, 1972a.

_____ and Associates. *The Dream Sellers.* San Francisco: Jossey-Bass, 1972b.

_____ and Associates. *Drug Dealers: Taking Action.* San Francisco: Jossey-Bass, 1973.

_____ and Associates Final Report of NIDA Grant No. DA 00097. *Drug Education: Impact and Outlook*. National Institute on Drug Abuse. Rockville, Maryland, 1975.

_____ and Ferguson, B. "Predicting Who Will Turn On." In: R.H. Blum and Associates. *Students and Drugs*. San Francisco: Jossey-Bass, 1970, pp. 278-288.

Boland, B. and Roizen, R. "Sales Slips and Survey Responses: New Data on the Reliability of Survey Consumption Measures." In: *The Drinking and Drug Practices Surveyor*, School of Public Health, University of California at Berkeley, August 1973, pp. 5-10.

Brazelton, T.B. "Effect of Prenatal Drugs on the Behavior of the Neorate." *American Journal of Psychiatry* 126 (1970): 95-100.

Brecher, E.M. and the Editors of Consumer Reports. *Licit and Illicit Drugs*. Mount Vernon, New York: Consumers Union, 1972.

Buder, L. "Students' Improved Behavior Laid to Drug-Prevention Drive." *New York Times* (Wednesday, April 26, 1973): 41.

Carney, R.E. *A Report on the Feasibility of Using Risk-Taking Attitudes as a Basis for Programs to Control and Predict Drug Abuse*. Coronado, Calif.: E.S.E.A. Title III Project, Coronado Unified School District, 1970a.

_____. *A Report on the Application of the Risk-Taking Attitude Questionnaire to the Fourth and Fifth Grades in the Coronado Unified School District*. Coronado, Calif.: E.S.E.A. Title III Project, 1970b.

_____. "Valuing and Drugs: Final, 1971-72, Report on the Tempe, Arizona, Drug Abuse Prevention Program." In: *Why Evaluate Drug Education? Report of a Task Force, May 1974, Enhancing Drug Education in the South*. Atlanta, Georgia: Southern Regional Education Board.

Cassel, R.N. and Zander, G. "Teach me What I Want to Know About Drugs for Junior High School Students." *The International Journal of the Addictions* 9 (1974): 541-567

Chein, L., Gerard, D.L., Lee, R.S., and Rosenfeld, E. *The Road to H: Narcotics, Delinquency and Social Policy*. New York: Basic Books, 1964.

Clark, J. (Director) "Operation Future: A Kings-Tulare Drug Abuse Control Project." Mimeograph. Courthouse, Visalia, Calif., Sept. 26, 1972.

Coleman, J.S., *et al. Equality of Educational Opportunity*. Washington, D.C.: U.S. Government Printing Office, 1966.

Cornacchia, H.J., Bentel, D.J., and Smith, D.E. *Drugs in the Classroom: A Conceptual Model for School Programs*. St. Louis: The C.V. Mosby Co., 1973.

Cowen, E.L. "Emergent Directions in School Mental Health." *American Scientist* 59 (Nov./Dec. 1971): 723-733.

Cox, T.J. and Longwell, B. "Reliability of Interview Data Concerning Current

Heroin Use from Heroin Addicts on Methadone." *The International Journal of the Addictions* 9 (1974): 161-165.

Crowdy, J.P. and Lewthwaite, C.J. "Smoking Habits of Young Soldiers. A Comparison between 1959 and 1966 Generations." *Journal of the Royal Army Medical Corps* 118 (1972): 168-172.

Cumming, E. and Cumming, J. *Closed Ranks: An Experiment in Mental Health Education*. Cambridge, Mass.: Harvard, 1957.

De Angelis, G.G. "Testing for Drugs—Advantages and Disadvantages." *The International Journal of the Addictions* 7 (1972): 365-385.

De Lone, R.H. "The Ups and Downs of Drug-Abuse Education." *Saturday Review of Education* (November 11, 1972): 27-32.

Dohner, V.A. "Alternatives to Drugs." *Addictions*. Addiction Research Foundation of Ontario (Fall 1972): 28-53.

Dorn, N. "Drug Education—Is It Effective?" *Drugs and Society* 1 (June 1972): 21-24.

Dunn, W.L., Jr., Ed. *Smoking Behavior: Motives and Incentives*. Washington, D.C.: V.H. Winston and Co., 1973.

Einstein, S., Lavenhar, M.A., Wolfson, E.A., Louria, D.B., Quinones, M.A., and Mc Ateer, G. "The Training of Teachers for Drug Abuse Education Programs: Preliminary Considerations." *Journal of Drug Education* 1(4) (Dec. 1971): 323-345.

Erickson, V.L. "Psychological Growth for Women: A Cognitive-Developmental Curriculum Intervention." *Counseling and Values* 18(2) (1974): 102-116.

Faber, Nancy. "Facts Alone Are Not Enough." *Learning* (Feb. 1973): 10-14.

Feinglass, S.J. "How to Plan a Drug Abuse Education Workshop." *Resource Book for Drug Abuse Education*, First and Second edition. Rockville, Maryland: National Clearinghouse for Drug Abuse Information, 1969, 1972.

Fejer, D. and Smart, R.G. "The Knowledge About Drugs, Attitudes Towards Them and Drug Use Rates of High School Students." *Journal of Drug Education* 3 (Winter 1973): 377-388.

Feldman, H. "Street Status and Drug Preference." In: V.L. Patch, ed. *Heroin Addiction*. Boston: Little Brown, 1972.

Finnish Foundation for Alcohol Studies and The European Regional Office of WHO. "Alcohol Control Policy and Public Health: Report on a Working Group." *The Drinking and Drug Practices Surveyor*, University of California Berkeley, School of Public Health (9) (Aug. 1974): 1, 32-39.

Gaber, I. "The Don'ts of Drug Surveys." *Drugs and Society*, London, England 1(10) (1972): 10-13.

Geis, G., Morgan, E.L., Schor, M., Bullington, B., and Munns, J.G. *Addicts in the Classroom: The Impact of an Experimental Narcotics Education Program on*

Junior High Pupils. Washington, D.C.: U.S. Office of Economic Opportunity, 1969. (Unpublished report.)

Girdano, D.A. and Girdano, D.D. *Drug Education: Content and Methods.* Reading, Mass.: Addison-Wesley Publishing Co., 1972.

Glenn, W.A. and Richards, L.G. *Recent Surveys of Non-Medical Drug Use: A Compendium of Abstracts.* Rockville, Maryland: National Institute on Drug Abuse, 1974.

Goldstein, J.W. "Getting High in High School: The Meaning of Adolescent Drug Usage." Paper presented to the American Ed. Research Association, New York, Feb., 1971. Report No. 71-3. Available from the Department of Psychology, Carnegie Mellon University, Pittsburgh, Pa.

_____. "Drug Education Worthy of the Name." *Impact: The Magazine for Innovation and Change in Counseling* 1 (1972): 18-24.

_____, Gleason, T.C., and Korn, J.H. "Whither the Epidemic? Psychoactive Drug-Use Career Patterns of College Students." *Journal of Applied Social Psychology* 5 (1975): 1.

Goodstadt, M.S. *Myths and Methodology in Drug Education: A Critical Review of The Research Evidence.* Substudy No. 588. Toronto, Canada: Addiction Research Foundation, 1974.

Haberman, P.W., Josephson, E., Zanes, A., and Elinson, J. "High School Drug Behavior: A Methodological Report on Pilot Studies." Paper presented to the First International Conference on Student Drug Surveys, Newark, New Jersey, Sept., 1971.

Hammond, P.G. As quoted in M. Korcok. "Drug Education Termed a 'Catastrophe'." *The Journal of The Addiction Research Foundation, Toronto, Canada* 1(6) (Nov, 1, 1972): 1.

Hampden, T. and Whitten, P. "Morals Left and Right." *Psychology Today* 4 (April 1971): 39-43, 74, 76.

Harlin, V.K. "The Influence of Obvious Anonymity on the Response of School Children to a Questionnaire About Smoking." *American Journal of Public Health* (April 1972): 566-574.

Hauser, R. "Prison Reform and Society." *Prison Service Journal* 3(9) (1963): 2-18.

Healy, P.F. and Manak, J.P., eds. *Drug Dependence and Abuse Resource Book.* Chicago, Illinois: National District Attorneys Association, 1971.

Hess, C.B. "Is There a Way Out of All This Drug Confusion?" *Pennsylvania's Health* 33 (Summer 1972): 16-24.

Illich, I. *Deschooling Society.* New York: Harper and Row, 1971.

Inkeles, A. "Becoming Modern: Individual Change in Six Developing Countries." *Ethos* 3 (1975): 323-342.

Imhof, J.E. *Drug Education for Teachers and Parents.* New York: William H. Sadlier, Inc., 1970.

Institute for the Study of Drug Dependence—Educational Research Unit. *Evaluation of Drug Education: Findings of a National Research Study of Effects on Secondary School Students of Five Types of Lesson Given by Teachers.* London, England: January, 1974.

Jellinek, E.M. *The Disease Concept of Alcoholism.* New Haven: Hillhouse, 1960.

Jencks, C. *et al. A Reassessment of the Effect of Family and Schooling in America.* New York: Basic Books, 1972.

Jenkins, C. "Value Characteristics of Ninth Grade Drug Abusers." Drug Prevention Program, Tempe Elementary District III, 1973. (Mimeograph.)

Jessor, R. and Jessor, S.L. "Adolescent Development and the Onset of Drinking: A Longitudinal Study." Institute of Behavioral Science, University of Colorado, May, 1974. (Monograph.)

Johnson, B.D. *Marijuana Users and Drug Subcultures.* New York: John Wiley and Sons, 1973.

Joint Commission on Mental Health of Children. *Crisis in Child Mental Health: Challenge for the 1970's.* New York: Harper and Row, 1969.

Joyce, C.R.B. "Some Possible Positive Reactions to Drug Abuse." *Society's Response.* London, England: Anglo-American Conference on Drug Abuse, April 16, 1973, pp. 32-36.

Judson, H.F. *Heroin Addiction in Britain.* New York: Harcourt, Brace, Jovanich, 1974.

Kandel, D.B. "Stages In Adolescent Involvement in Drug Use." *Science* 190 (1975): 912-914.

_____ and Lesser, G.S. *Youth in Two Worlds.* San Francisco: Jossey-Bass, Inc., 1972.

Kay, WM. *Moral Education.* Hamden, Conn.: Linnet Books, The Shoe String Press, Inc., 1975.

Kinder, B.N. "Attitudes Toward Alcohol and Drug Abuse. II. Experimental Data, Mass Media Research, and Methodological Considerations." *International Journal of the Addictions* 10 (1975): 1035-1054.

Kleber, H.D., Berberian, R.M., Gould, L.C., and Kasl, S.V. *Evaluation of an Adolescent Drug Education Program.* Final Report, NIDA Grant No. DA-00055. Yale University School of Medicine, New Haven, Connecticut, May, 1975.

Kohlberg, L. "The Development of Children's Orientations Toward a Moral Order. II. Social Experience, Social Conduct, and the Development of Moral Thought." *Vita Humana.* IX. (1966).

Kurzman, T. "A Non-Drug Approach to Drug Education." *Addictions,* Addiction Research Foundation of Ontario (Summer 1974): 50-63.

Lawler, J.T. "Peer Group Approach to Drug Education." *Journal of Drug Education* 1(1) (March 1971): 63-76.

Leonard, G. *Education and Ecstasy*. New York: Delacorte Press, 1968.

Lipp. M., Tinklenberg, J., Taintor, Z. *et al.* "Marijuana Use Among Students at Four U.S. Medical Schools." Paper presented at the Second World Meeting on Medical Law, Washington, D.C., August 18, 1970.

Love, L.R. and Kaswan, J.W. *Troubled Children: Their Families, Schools and Treatments*. New York: John Wiley and Sons, 1974.

Luetgert, M.J. and Armstrong, A.H. "Methodological Issues in Drug Usage Surveys: Anonymity, Recency and Frequency." *International Journal of the Addictions* 8 (1973): 683-689.

Mason, M.L. *Drug Education Effects: Final Report* (Young Adult Services, Gainesville, Fla.). Washington, D.C.: National Center for Educational Research and Development, March 1972.

Michigan Department of Education. *Drug Education Guidelines*. Lansing, Michigan: 1973.

Miller, Martin. "Drug Education: A Re-evaluation." *Journal of Drug Education* 1 (March 1971): 15-24.

Montalvo, J.G., Scrignar, C.B., Alderette, E., Harper, B., and Eyer, D. "Flushing, Pale-Colored Urines, and False Negatives—Urinalysis of Narcotic Addicts." *The International Journal of the Addictions* 7 (1972): 355-364.

Mussen, P., Langer, J., and Covington, M. *New Directions in Developmental Psychology*. New York: Holt, Rinehart and Winston, 1969.

National Clearinghouse for Drug Abuse Information.*Selected Drug Education Curricula Series*. Superintendent of Documents, U.S. Government Printing Office, Washington, D.C., 1970.

_____. *Resource Book for Drug Abuse Education, Second Edition*. Superintendent of Documents, U.S. Government Printing Office, 1972.

National Institute of Mental Health. *For the Parents of a Young Child: Tips on Drug Abuse Prevention*. Superintendent of Documents, U.S. Government Printing Office, Washington, D.C., 1972.

Nettler, G. *Explaining Crime*. New York: McGraw Hill, 1974.

Niemi, R.G. *How Family Members Perceive Each Other: Political and Social Attitudes in Two Generations*. New Haven, Conn.: Yale University Press, 1974.

North Allegheny School District. *Human Growth and Development Curriculum*. Pittsburgh, Pa.: 1971.

Office of Education. "Alcohol and Drug Education Program. III. Prevention and Education," Washington, D.C., 1975. (Mimeograph.)

Parry, H., Balter, M., and Cisin, I. "Primary Levels of Underreporting Psycho-tropic Drug Use." *Public Opinion Quarterly* 34 (1970-71): 582-592.

Payne, J. "No Help for the Young." *Drugs and Society* 1(1) (1971): 8-11.

Petzel, T.P., Johnson, J.E., and Mc Killip, J. "Response Bias in Drug Surveys." *Journal of Consulting and Clinical Psychology* 40(3) (1973): 437-439.

Piaget, J. *The Moral Judgment of the Child.* New York: Free Press, 1965. (Originally printed in 1932.)

Pichot, P., Buchsenschutz, E., and Perse, J. *Simposio Droga E Societa Off. E Domai.* Milan, Italy: Museo Nazionale Della Scienza E Della Tecnica, October 1972.

Poliakoff, M. "Training 'Turned-On' Health Teachers." *Journal of Drug Education* 1(2) (June 1971): 187-193.

Robins, L.N. *Deviant Children Grown Up.* Baltimore, Maryland: The Williams and Wilkins Co., 1966.

_____ and Guze, S.B. "Drinking Practices and Problems in Urban Ghetto Populations." In: *Recent Advances in Studies of Alcoholism.* Superintendent of Documents, Department of HEW, U.S. Government Printing Office, 1972, pp. 825-842.

Roser, M. "The Role of Schools in Heading off Delinquency." Cited in: S. Rubin. *Crime and Juvenile Delinquency.* Dobbs Ferry, New York: Oceana Publications, 1970.

Rubin, S. *Crime and Juvenile Delinquency.* Dobbs Ferry, New York: Oceana Publications, Inc., 1970.

San Mateo County Survey. *Preliminary Summary–1973, San Mateo County, Calif., Surveillance of Student Drug Use.* San Mateo, Calif.: Department of Health and Welfare, 1973.

Schaps, E., Sanders, C., and Hughes, P. *District 214 Drug Survey: An Interim Report.* Department of Psychiatry, University of Chicago, June 1971.

Schmidt, W. Cited in: B. Boland and R. Roizen. "Sales Slips and Survey Responses: New Data on the Reliability of Survey Consumption Measures." *The Drinking and Drug Practices Surveyor* No. 8, School of Public Health, University of California at Berkeley (August 1973): 5-10.

Schwartz, D.J. "Let's Hear It One More Time." Speech delivered to Experience '74 Conference at Canada College, sponsored by the San Mateo County Office of Education, June 1974. (Mimeograph.)

Schwilk, G.L. "An Experimental Study of the Effectiveness of Direct and Indirect Methods of Character Education." *Union College Student Character Education* 1 (1956): 199-229.

Segal, Mark. "Drug Education: Toward a Rational Approach." *The International Journal of the Addictions* 7(2) (1972): 257-284.

Slimmon, Lee. "Alternatives and Values Clarification." Annual Report, County of Marin, July 10, 1973. (Mimeograph.)

Smart, R.G. "Sources of Drug Information for High School Students: Their Relative Influence and Credibility." *Journal of Alcohol Education* 17 (1971): 1-15.

_____ and Fejer, D. *Drug Education: Current Issues, Future Directions.* Toronto: Addiction Research Foundation of Ontario, 1974.

_____ and Jackson, D. Cited in: P.C. Whitehead and R.G. Smart. "Validity and Reliability of Self-Reported Drug Use." *Canadian Journal of Criminology and Corrections*, Ottawa, Canada 14(1) (January 1972): 1-7.

Smith, G.M. "Rebellious Behavior Predicts Drug Use." As reported in *The Social Seminar Newsletter SCAN*, July 1973, p. 8.

Smith, Gene M. and Lindemann, E. "Antecedents of Teenage Drug Use." Department of Psychiatry, Massachusetts General Hospital, Boston, Mass. (Undated mimeograph, circa 1973.)

Stamford Board of Education, Stamford Public Schools, Conn. *Stamford Curriculum Guide for Drug Abuse Education.* Stamford, Conn.: 1971.

State of Ohio Department of Education, Dayton City Board of Education, and Educational Research Council of America. *A World To Grow In.* Cleveland, Ohio: 1972.

Stevenson, H.W. *Children's Learning.* New York: Appleton-Century-Crofts, 1972.

Stuart, R.B. "Teaching Facts About Drugs: Pushing or Preventing." *Journal of Educational Psychology* 66(2) (April 1974): 189-201.

Swisher, J.D., and Hoffman, A.M. "Real Research in Drug Education. Drug Information: The Irrelevant Variable." Paper presented at American Personnel and Guidance Association Convention, Atlantic City, New Jersey, April, 1971.

_____ and Horan, J.J. "Effecting Drug Attitude Change in College Students via Induced Cognitive Dissonance." Reported by M. Goodstadt in: *Myths and Methodology in Drug Education: A Critical Review of the Research Evidence*, Substudy No. 588. Toronto, Canada: Addiction Research Foundation, 1974.

_____ and Horman, R.E. "Drug Abuse Prevention." Reported by M. Goodstadt in: *Myths and Methodology in Drug Education: A Critical Review of the Research Evidence*, Substudy No. 588. Toronto, Canada: Addiction Research Foundation, 1974.

_____ and Piniuk, A.J. "An Evaluation of Keystone Central School District's Drug Education Program." Reported by M. Goodstadt in: *Myths and Methodology in Drug Education: A Critical Review of the Research Evidence*, Substudy No. 588. Toronto, Canada: Addiction Research Foundation, 1974. (Mimeograph.)

_____ and Warner, R.W. *A Study of Four Approaches to Drug Abuse Prevention*, Final Report, Project No. OB 083. Washington, D.C.: U.S. Department of HEW, Office of Education, Bureau of Research, Region III, July 3, 1971.

Tresan, D.I. "An Experimental Drug Education Program in the San Francisco City Schools." San Francisco: Langley Porter Neuropsychiatric Institute. (Undated manuscript, circa 1972.)

Turiel, E. "Developmental Processes in Child's Moral Thinking." In: P. Mussen, J. Langer and M. Covington, eds. *New Directions in Developmental Psychology*. New York: Holt, Rinehart and Winston, 1969.

Universal Research Systems, Inc. *Drug Decision*, Fourth edition. Sunnyvale, Calif.: Universal Research Systems, Inc., 1971.

U.S. Department of Health, Education and Welfare, Public Health Service. *Adult Use of Tobacco*. Washington, D.C.: National Clearinghouse for Smoking and Health, June, 1973.

U.S. Department of Transportation. *Alcohol and Alcohol Safety*, 3 vols: K-6, Junior High, and Senior High. Washington, D.C.: Superintendent of Documents, U.S. Government Printing Office, 1973.

U.S. Office of Education, "Alcohol and Drug Education Program. III. Prevention and Education, Washington, D.C., 1975. (Mimeograph.)

Visco, E.P. and Finotti, J.F. *Spark Program Analysis, Final Report.* Washington, D.C.: Geomet Report No. HF-347, 1974.

Weaver, S.C. and Tennant, F.S., Jr. "Effectiveness of Drug Education Programs for Secondary School Students." *American Journal of Psychiatry* 130(7) (July 1973): 812-814.

Wechsler, H. and Thom, D. *Alcohol and Drug Use Among Teenagers: A Questionnaire Study.* Paper prepared for the Second Annual Alcoholism Conference, National Institute of Alcohol Abuse and Alcoholism, Washington, D.C., June 1, 1972.

Weil, A.T. "Altered States of Consciousness." In: The Drug Abuse Council. *Dealing with Drug Abuse*. New York: Praeger, 1972, pp. 329-344.

Whitehead, P.C. and Brook, P. Cited in: P.C. Whitehead and R.G. Smart. "Validity and Reliability of Self-Reported Drug Use." *Canadian Journal of Criminology and Correction*, Ottawa, Canada 14(1) (January 1972).

_____ and Smart, R.G. "Validity and Reliability of Self-Reported Drug Use." *Canadian Journal of Criminology and Correction*, Ottawa, Canada 14(1) (January 1972).

Woodcock, J. "Action in the Schools." In: R.H. Blum and Associates. *Drug Dealers: Taking Action*. San Francisco: Jossey-Bass, 1973, pp. 267-281.

World Health Organization, Expert Committee on Drug Dependence. Technical Report Series 460, Eighteenth Report, Geneva, 1970.

_____. Technical Report Series 551, Twentieth Report, Geneva, 1974.

Yolles, S.F. "Prescription for Drug Abuse Education: Managing the Mood Changers." *Journal of Drug Education* 1 (June 1971): 101-113.

Zajonc, R. "Brainwash: Familiarity Breeds Comfort." *Psychology Today* 3(9) (February 1970): pp. 32-35, 60-62.

Zinberg, N.E., Boris, H.N., and Boris, M. *Teaching Social Change.* Baltimore: Johns Hopkins University Press, 1976.

Index

Index

Abrams, L.A., 8n, 51
Abruzzi, D. and Abruzzi, W., 21
Absences, excessive, 104-109, 112, 118, 120-121, 148
Absenteeism, 23, 55, 104, 113, 144
Abstainers versus users, 71, 78-79, 115-118, 121-122
Abstinence syndrome from drugs, 6-7, 11, 59, 83-84, 96-97, 139, 169, 174; total, 3, 58, 176
Academic: competition, 107; education and subjects, 121, 145, 149-150, 164; performance, 18
Accidents, 1, 6, 12, 17, 183; home, 58; prevention of, 4; road and traffic, 31, 58, 97
Accountability in Drug Education (Abrams), 8n, 51
Achievement levels, 144, 156, 162
Activism and activity ratings, 21, 46
Addiction and addicts, 11, 60, 97, 153, 176
Adjustments, 20; difficulties in, 36; personal, 10, 111, 113, 120; social, 29, 113; vocational, 28
Administrative control and support, 94, 97, 100, 102, 149-150
Administrators, school, 1, 5, 7, 17, 40, 99, 108, 111, 133, 139, 148, 184, 189
Adulthood, 37, 136, 175
Adventurism, spirit of, 39
Advertising, results of, 29
Aerosol sprays, 82, 125
Age levels, factor of, 7-8, 14-17, 45, 48-49, 63, 65, 73, 82, 91, 97, 113, 117, 119, 125, 131, 135, 163-164, 174-175, 183, 187, 189
Agencies: community, 8, 41, 45, 55, 186; family service, 185, 188; mental health, 113; referral to, 100, 104-109, 112-113, 121; service, 112-113, 121; state education, 41

Aggressiveness, drug-related, 3, 101
Agricultural areas, 14
Airplane glue, 125
Ahlstrom, W.M., 28
Alcohol, problems and use of, 2, 5-7, 10, 13, 15, 18, 29, 31, 33, 48, 53, 69, 71, 75, 77, 79, 83-84, 95, 110, 115, 119, 129, 131, 149, 153, 157, 176, 186-187
Alcoholics and alcoholism, 3, 11, 22, 53-54, 58, 96, 153-154, 159
Alertness, 6
Alienation, mood of, 19, 39-40
Alternative nonspecific activities and satisfactions, 34, 39, 45, 55, 65, 96-97, 177, 187
American Cancer Society, 53
American School Health Association, 46
Amorality, 39
Amphetamines: prevalence levels of, 80, 82-83; use of, 3, 7, 10, 12, 15-16, 24, 31, 54, 58, 61, 71-72, 75, 77, 110, 128-129, 187n
Antagonism, mood of, 21, 36, 134
Antiasthmatics, 125
Anticigarette education, 53
Antidemocratic social views, 122
Antidepressant drugs, 15, 18, 119
Antidrug effects, 52
Antischool attitudes, 22-23
Antisocial activities, 21
Anxiety, 31, 47, 53, 114, 183
Apathy, classroom, 21, 173
Aptitudes, classroom, 5, 165-166
Armstrong, A.H., 59
Arrests, drug incurred, 2, 11-12, 16-17, 29, 83, 97
Attendance problems and records, 56, 100-110, 121, 144-150, 165-166
Attention span, decrease in, 47
Attitudes: acceptance of, 135; antidrug, 52; antischool, 22-23; changes

Attitudes *(continued)*
in, 51-52; children's, 47, 155;
home, 158; importance of, 19-20,
32, 34, 66; liberalization of, 53;
permissive, 49; positive, 102; self,
100; sets of, 2, 10; students', 148;
teachers', 151; tolerant, 57; work
and play, 43
Australia, 32
Authoritarianism, 35, 147
Authority, 17, 138, 145; derogating,
146; of father, 153; juvenile, 186;
legal, 185; medical, 185; probation,
188; response to, 150; school, 114,
176, 185-186
Automobile and highway, 31, 58, 97
Autonomy, 37, 43, 136

Background, 66; children's, 63-64;
economic, 152; educational, 19;
family, 119, 122; impoverished, 12;
socioeconomic, 149, 165; student's,
149-150
Bad: companions, 27; outcomes, 2, 7,
11-12, 22; trips, 16-17, 51n
Barbiturates, use of, 3, 5, 7, 10, 15-16,
23, 29, 54, 71-72, 75, 77, 80-83,
110, 115, 128-129, 145, 187n
Becker, Howard, 9
Bedworth, A.E., 34, 46
Beer, consumption of, 31, 61n, 71-72,
154, 164
Behavior: aberrant, 36; changes in,
109; conventional, 174; delinquent,
113; destructive, 40; deviant, 25;
drinking, 18; drug induced, 29,
158; interpersonal, 3; personal, 5;
problems in, 39, 100, 104-107,
110, 113, 121, 123; standard for,
155; superficial, 56
Benefits, 8, 29-30
Berberian, R.M., 54, 171
Beverages, 77, 95. *See also specific
type of beverage*
Biochemical reactions, 9, 12, 174
Biological rhythms and essays, 15,
60-61, 95

Birdwood, G., 33
Birk, E., 26
Blacks and the black community, 22,
144-145, 149, 162, 165
Blum and Associates, 11, 29, 31-33,
59-61, 66, 68n, 96, 114, 121, 149,
154
Boards of Education, 7
Boland, B., 58
Boredom, mood of, 36, 39-40, 162-
163
Boyle Heights study, 48, 54
Brazelton, T.B., 95
Brecher, E.M., 53
Brook, P., 59
Buder, L., 55
Budgets and budgeting, 7, 59
Bureaucracy and bureaucrats, 27, 33,
43

California, surveys in, 14, 23, 28-29,
48, 54, 61, 63, 67n, 75, 82, 84-85,
95, 133, 169, 174-176
Canada, students in, 47-49
Cancer, 53; lung, 3, 31
Cannabis, use of, 10, 14-18, 23, 28-31,
61n, 171, 185
Capitalism, 176
Career considerations, 36
Carney, R.E., 34, 54
Cassel, R.N., 49
Census data, 94
Certification, demand for, 27
Change patterns, 86-91, 100-101, 111,
121, 129, 137-138
Character: building, 43; defects, 102,
104, 105, 109, 112, 121; disorders,
15; education, 4, 42-44
Chemicals, 4, 15
Chicago, surveys in, 48-49
Child care facilities, 32, 183, 189
Child rearing and guidance, 56, 66,
116-117, 119-122, 152, 156, 170-
171, 175
"Chippers," heroin, 17
Choice, freedom of, 35, 97
Church, influence of, 47-48, 115, 139,
176

Cigarettes, consumption of, 5-6, 11, 16, 29, 33, 58-59, 77, 82, 154, 156, 164, 185, 187n
Cirrhosis of the liver, 3, 12
Civic obligations, 3
Clark, J., 34
Classification system, 23, 86-87, 106, 111, 117-118, 121, 125, 129
Classroom grade levels: second, 14, 17, 63-65, 73-74, 77, 79, 99, 102-103, 120, 133, 137-139, 169; third, 65, 77, 138, 169; fourth, 17, 21, 54, 63-66, 69-70, 73-77, 82-85, 88, 91-92, 98, 102-104, 120-121, 127, 129, 131-139, 172; fifth, 21, 65, 74, 77, 79, 82, 98, 137-138, 140-141; sixth, 14, 17, 21, 54, 63-66, 69-70, 73-77, 82-85, 88, 91-92, 98, 103-106, 113, 120-121, 125, 127, 129-133, 137-143, 152, 172, 174; seventh, 21, 28, 48, 50, 53, 63, 74-77, 85, 98, 125, 137-138, 140, 171-172; eighth, 21, 28, 50, 53-54, 63-70, 74-75, 77, 79, 82-85, 91-92, 98, 102, 120-121, 125, 127, 130-134, 137-143, 156, 159, 171-172; ninth, 21, 53, 77n, 83, 85, 98, 102, 169-171; tenth, 21, 63-64, 73, 75, 77-78, 85-88, 91, 97, 99, 105-111, 120-121, 127-130, 133, 169, 171; eleventh, 21, 77-78, 83, 107, 134, 143, 159, 169; twelfth, 21, 85, 169
Class sizes, importance of, 93-95
Clerical records, 100
Clinical observations, 49-50, 66-67, 143-144, 161, 172, 189
Clinics, drug, 59, 184
Cocaine, use of, 7, 16, 54, 71-72, 77, 81-83, 97, 110, 115, 129, 187n
Coffee, stimulation of, 2, 6, 15-16
Coleman, J.S., 19
College: drug use in, 21n, 96; professors, 18; students, 46, 48, 59, 61, 114
Coma, lapse into, 3
Communication: interpersonal, 39; need for, 40-41, 55, 175; resources, 34; skills, 34; spiritual, 31

Community: agencies, 8, 41, 45, 55, 186; centers, 31; involvement, 55, 184; leaders, 1, 149; milieu differences, 151, 166, 171; norms, 27, 175; programs, 85, 184; prohibitions, 174; resources, 45, 188; spirit, 43; values, 167; workshop, 40
Competition, academic, 113, 162
Computer printouts and records, 99-100, 108
Conduct: problems of, 19, 108, 113, 121, 183; social, 156, 172
Confidentiality, requirement of, 65, 70
Conformity, forces of, 35-36, 152, 173
Connecticut, 54, 171
Conscience, voice of, 27, 155-156
Consciousness, state of, 30-31, 135-136
Conservatism, philosophy of, 122, 135, 141, 177
Constraints, 50, 96, 136
Consumer protection and satisfaction, 68, 133, 142, 174, 189
Control: delinquency, 185-187; of drugs, 25; governmental, 7; group, 28-29, 50, 52, 56, 67, 85, 89-91, 93, 95-98, 135; school, 134; social, 170, 186; teacher, 152
Conventionality, philosophy of, 3-4, 18, 130, 149
Coordination, lack of, 55
Cornacchia, H.J., 46
Costs and benefit analysis, 2, 176
Counseling and counselors: casework, 56; family, 40; group, 30, 52-53; pastoral, 185; professional, 55; role of, 5, 49, 139, 184; school, 1, 49, 55; services, 28-29, 34-35; youth, 39, 41, 45
Course loads taken, 107, 110
Cowen, E.L., 36
Cox, T.J., 59-60
Credibility, source, 48-49
Crime, 30, 149; victimless, 185; violent, 186

Criminal law, 19, 28
"Crisis" intervention, 189
Crowdy, J.P., 58n
Culture: as alternative, 55; factor and influence of, 15, 22-23, 30, 54, 58, 120; patterns of, 11, 13; resources, 39; school, 35; value of, 3, 6
Cummings, E. and Cummings, J., 33
Curiosity, element of, 158-159
Curriculum development and planning, 40, 43, 55, 68, 133, 135, 141, 170-173, 190

DeAngelis, G.G., 60
Death and fear of dying, 3, 18, 36, 98, 163, 176
Decentralization, federal role in, 2
Decisions and decision-making, 26, 34-35, 37, 140, 156, 167, 169; conscious, 38-39, 134-136; rational, 45
Decriminalization of drug use, 52
D'Elia, J.A., 34, 46
Delinquents and delinquencies, 1, 4, 14-16, 19-22, 25, 28-29, 36, 42, 100, 102, 105, 109, 112, 121, 149, 165, 170, 173, 177, 183-187
Delirium tremens, 11
DeLone, R.H., 35-36, 38
Democratic procedures, 14, 43, 157
Dental hygiene, 25, 52
Depression and depressants, 18, 61n, 184
Destabilization, 98
Detoxification centers, 185
Deviant: behavior, 25, 173; drug use, 21, 164
Didactic classroom education, 30, 36-37, 52, 67, 74, 85, 88-91, 93-97, 130, 132, 134, 136, 156, 165-166, 170, 172, 189-190
Disadvantaged homes, 28, 43, 162
Discipline: child, 116-117; internal, 13; parental, 12, 155; problems of, 43, 55, 121, 139, 144, 159, 162; social, 24; students, 150
Discrimination, 104-105, 109-111, 117-118, 132, 171

Discussion groups, 40, 137, 140, 166, 171
Disease, drug-related, 6. *See also specific illnesses*
Divorces, prevalence of, 115-116, 149
Dohner, V.A., 34, 36
Domicile status, 104-105
"Dope," 154
Dorn, N., 48
Dream Sellers, The (Blum and Associates), 31
Drinking habits: high school, 21-23; patterns and problems of, 18, 41, 54, 70, 95, 153, 161, 165; preteen, 12; social, 13; unsupervised, 29, 31
Drop-in centers, 40
Dropouts, 17, 21, 40, 64, 100, 145, 164
Drug Abuse Council, 51
Drug Dealers Taking Action (Richard Blum and Associates), 33n
Drug Education: Impact and Outlook (Grant), 68n
Drug Prevention Branch of the Office of Education, 188
Drugs: abuse of, 2-3; dealers in, 25, 29, 31, 33, 176; demonology of, 26-27; education in, 2-3, 25-27, 43-45, 57, 63, 82-98, 173-174; fictitious, 52, 59; treatment centers, 188; unknown, 58; use patterns of, 10, 62, 170-171
Drunkenness, 97, 164, 185. *See also* Alcoholics and alcoholism

Economic forces, 2, 16
Education and Ecstasy (Leonard), 36
Education, Boards of, 41
Education, Departments of, 34, 41, 46
Education, impact of, 4, 17, 19, 25, 38, 42-47, 50-58, 83, 130-131
Education, Office of, 39, 42, 45, 56, 189
Educational Research Council of America, 46
Edwards, Griffith, 42
Efficiency, disadvantage of, 7
Egalitarianism, 175

Einstein, S., 34
Elementary schools, 20, 42, 62-63, 66, 83, 85, 94-97, 102n, 114, 116, 134-135, 140-141, 147-150, 166, 169, 171
Elitism, 44
Emergency cases, drug, 55
Emotions and emotionalism, 5, 12, 30, 37, 45, 47-50, 113, 144, 164, 186
England, 27, 48, 52
Enjoyment, class, 133-134
Environment: factor of, 2, 28, 33, 83, 95; family, 20; home, 117, 144; school, 6, 8, 143; social, 4, 39
Epidemiology, 9, 14, 188
Erickson, V.L., 42
Errors and inaccuracies, 71-73, 101, 125, 127-128
Escapism, 4
Ethics, context of, 27, 30, 38
Ethnic groups, 11, 13, 100, 110, 114, 121, 152, 184
Etiology of drug use, 9, 15, 18, 30, 35, 122, 175
European Regional Office of World Health Organization, 54
Evaluation: degrees of, 32-33, 141, 166; family, 66; parents, 140; research, 41
Excitement, mood of, 21
Exotic drugs, 31
Experience, personal and social, 141, 169
Experimentation, 16, 61, 91, 97, 132, 159
Expert Committee on Drug Dependence of World Health Organization, 26, 35
Exploitation, 39

Failure, fear of, 40
Family, the, 2, 15, 45, 47, 66, 174, 190; attributes, 111, 120; background, 118-119, 122; conventional, 149; counseling, 40-41; discord, 4, 7, 22, 39, 170; features, 113, 122; income, 12, 23, 48, 108, 150; independence from, 36; influence,

58, 114-120, 151, 159, 166; instability, 117; liberal, 183; life, 10-11, 22, 143; planning courses, 34; problems, 103-106; status, 66, 99-100, 108-110; studies, 30-31, 116, 118; training, 18-20; values, 66, 170
Father: absence of, 11; authority of, 153; occupation of, 100, 103, 105, 109; values of, 119
Fatigue retarded performance, 3, 146
Federal Drug Enforcement Administration, 189
Federal government role, 2, 39
Federal Trade Commission, 162
Feinglass, S.J., 34
Fejer, D., 49, 52, 57, 59
Feldman, H., 38
Ferguson, B., 61
Field trips, school, 55
Fights and fighting, 18, 147
Films, shock, 48, 51, 161, 163
Financial resources, 39, 41
Finnish Foundation for Alcohol Studies, 54
Finotti, J.F., 45, 55
Foresightedness, need for, 42-43
France, 11, 96
Freud, Sigmund, 27
Friends, 11, 47, 138
Frustration, mood of, 40
Fundamentalist religious background, 12
Funds, appropriation of, 27

Gaber, I., 58
Garfield, E.F., 8n
Gary, Indiana, 56
Gasoline, 11, 71n, 82, 125
Geis, G., 48, 54
Generation gap, 19
Genetic features, 9, 12
Geography, factor of, 14, 32
Germany, 149
Ghetto, problems of, 22-23
Girdano, D.A. and Girdano, D.D., 46
Glenn, W.A., 85
Glue, sniffing of, 3, 11, 29, 71n, 82, 125, 127

Goals: clarification of, 3, 8, 20-21, 32, 35, 42, 114; educational, 38, 82; parental, 140, student, 164; teaching, 38

Goldstein, J.W., 10, 46, 48, 61, 71

Goodstadt, M.S., 51, 56

Grade levels, 7, 55, 89-93, 134-135, 144, 165-166. *See also* Classroom grade levels

Grade schools, 14, 17

Graduate students, 14, 71

Greek heritage, 13, 147

Group interaction sessions, 30, 37-38, 40, 55, 137, 140, 166, 171

Guttman scale, 71-72

Guze, S.B., 22-23

Haberman, P.W., 59

Hair sprays, 71n

Hallucinogens, 7, 14-16, 54, 61n, 71-72, 77, 82, 110, 128-129, 184, 187n

Hammond, P.G., 33

Hampden, T., 42

Hard drugs, 7. *See also specific type of hard drugs*

Harlin, V.K., 59

Harlow Elementary School, 144, 148-149

Hauser, R., 28

Havighurst, R.S., 28

Health: education, 2, 54; hazards, 29, 177, 183; infants and childs, 119, 183; personnel, 1; problems of, 20, 28, 66, 83, 113-114, 121, 189. *See also* Mental health

Health Education Council of the United Kingdom, 26

Health, Education and Welfare, Department of, 95, 189

Healy, P.F., 46

Heart disease, 3, 31, 53

Hedonism, 4, 17

Hepatitis, needle induced, 3, 97

Heroin, 5, 9, 11, 14, 16-18, 21, 24, 38-39, 54, 58, 60, 71-72, 75, 77, 81-82, 97, 115, 129, 154

High risk drug use, 107, 109-110, 112, 120, 172, 183-184, 190

High schools, 10, 14, 17, 19-20, 23, 42, 48, 50, 55, 59, 63-64, 67-71, 75, 83, 95-96, 106, 114, 125, 133-134, 137-138, 166; Junior, 21, 49-52, 54, 85; Senior, 21, 54, 85

Hippies, 14, 31

Hispanic students, 110

Hobbies, need for, 118

Hoffman, A.M., 52

Holland, 32

Home, the: accidents in, 58; disadvantaged, 43; environment, 117, 144; moral teaching in, 157; privileged, 43n; relationships, 35, 104-105; visits, 55, 143, 146

Homicides, 29

Hoodlumism, 147

Horan, J.J., 54

Horatio Alger's Children (Blum and Associates), 114, 119, 122

Horman, R.E., 54

Hospitals, 55, 164

Households, addiction prone, 2, 152-153

Humanism and human resources, 35-36, 41, 43

Humor, lack of, 12

Hyperactive, drug-induced, 184

Identity, 37, 39

Ideology, political, 17, 176

Illegitimacy, 149

Illich, Ivan, 43, 45

Illicit substances and use of, 1-2, 8, 10, 14-15, 19, 21, 26, 28, 30, 48, 53, 57-58, 70, 96, 109, 117, 119, 121, 176, 185, 187

Illnesses, drug or smoking induced, 11, 18, 28, 83, 97, 173

Imhof, J.E., 46

Immigrants, 149, 164

Immorality, 3, 50

Impulsiveness, 39, 42

Inattentiveness, trait of, 164-165

Income: and drinking habits, 12;

family, 12, 23, 48, 108, 150; levels of, 17, 94, 120, 184
Inconsistency rate, 73-76, 127-128
Independence, value of, 18-19, 36, 42, 159
Indoctrination, social, 37
Infections, contracting of, 17, 31, 184
Information: adequacy of, 63; dissemination of, 40, 53; distortion of, 174; source preferences of, 48, 52; technical, 157
Inhalants and use of, 3, 11, 14-15, 24, 71-72, 82-85, 125-132, 187n
Injectables, 54, 77, 83, 97, 110, 187
Inkeles, A., 94n
Instability: emotional, 12, 164; family, 117; periods of, 82, 84, 86, 189
Institute for the Study of Drug Dependence (London), 48, 51
Intellectual ability, 21, 43, 47, 55, 165
Interest-crafts, 103-110
Interests: personal, 120; professional, 141; stimulation of, 53, 65-66, 100-101, 172; vested, 27, 32
Interpersonal relations, 45
Interracial friction, 147
Intervention techniques, 42, 77, 82, 87, 91, 175, 189
Interviews: clinical, 161; end-of-study, 99, 104; family, 66, 68; parents, 66, 151; personal and confidential, 60, 74-75, 116, 144, 146-148, 155, 166, 184; retest procedures, 71; with teachers, 111
Intoxicants, volatile, 71n, 125
Investigations, local, 3
Irrationality, age of, 175
Italian heritage, 13, 147, 149, 159

Jackson, D., 59
Jails and imprisonment, 19, 164
James, William, 31
Jellinek, E.M., 95
Jencks, C., 19
Jenkins, C., 21
Jessor, R. and Jessor, S.L., 10, 18, 21
Jewish heritage, 13

Johnson, B.D., 21
Joint Commission on Mental Health of Children, 32
Joyce, C.R.B., 53
Judgment, 42, 190; independent, 159; moral, 30, 33; poor, 15
Judson, H.F., 42
Juniper High School, 144, 147-152, 159, 164
Junkies, 14
Juvenile authorities, 40, 113, 185-188

Kandel, D.B., 10, 19, 61, 71
Kaswan, J.W., 19, 21
Kay, William M., 43-45
Kinde, Mrs., school teacher, 144-146, 161-162, 165
Kinder, B.N., 57
Kindergarten, 34, 138
Kleber, H.D., 54
Kohlberg, L., 42
Kurzman, T., 34

Labor unions, 114
Language skills, 60, 146
Law and order, respect for, 116-117
Lawfulness, 43n, 162
Lawler, J.T., 46, 49
Laws, 25, 28, 32, 40, 134, 139
Leaders and leadership: governmental, 39; group, 37, 55; role of, 100-101, 104-106, 110, 112, 186; training, 39-41
Learning, awareness of, 109-110, 135, 143
Lectures, 119
Legal aid and authorities, 34, 40, 185
Legislation, drug, 17, 25
Leisure time, 108, 115, 119, 122
Leonard, George, 36
Lesser, G.S., 19
Lewthwaite, C.J., 58
Liberalism, 11
Libertarian trends, 175
Lieberman Research, Inc., 53
Life styles, 3, 10, 14, 20, 35, 167, 185
Lipp, M., 49

Liquor, 61n, 71-72, 82. *See also* Alcohol
Literature: children's, 47; medical, 3; scientific, 46, 120
Liver, damage to, 3, 12
Loneliness, feeling of, 39
Longwell, B., 59-60
Love, L.R., 19,21
Love, lack of, 12
LSD, use of, 3, 5, 10, 14, 16-17, 31, 48, 53, 58, 72, 75, 83
Luetgert, M.J., 59

Maladjustments, 29-30
Manak, J.P., 46
Manson "family," 31
Marijuana, use of, 2-7, 10-11, 14-15, 18-19, 22-23, 48, 52-53, 58-59, 70-72, 75-78, 82, 87, 101, 107-112, 115-117, 120, 129, 131, 153, 159, 187
Marimba High School, 144-152, 155, 157, 161-165
Marital stability, 115, 121; separation, 116, 149
Mason, M.L., 52
Mass media, 48-49
Massachusetts, 50
Measurement, question of, 58-62
Medical: authorities, 185; care, 25; experimentation, 61; films, 51n; literature, 3; patients, 60; practice, 10; students, 49
Medicines and medication, 3-4, 184; over-the-counter, 2, 15; self, 4, 18
Meditation, 31, 40
Meher Baba, 30-31
Mental health, 4-5, 15, 17, 27-28, 34, 36, 45, 49, 113, 117, 158, 184-185, 188
Mescaline, 72
Methadone maintenance program, 16, 60
Metropolitan centers, 12, 14
Mexican-Americans, 48, 147
Michigan, 34, 53
Middle class living, 14-17, 21, 145, 148-149, 162

Miller, Martin, 46
Mind, state of, 2
Mind Benders, film, 161
Minnesota Survey, 49
Minority groups, 12, 176
Misuse of Drugs Act in United Kingdom, 25-26
Monoamytriplamate (MOT), 52, 59
Montalvo, J.G., 60
Moods and mood elevators, 2, 16, 36
Moral soundness, 1, 3, 5, 7, 26, 30, 33-36, 42-44, 50, 136, 156-157, 167, 172, 176-177, 189
Morality, principles of, 30, 37, 42, 45, 157, 174
Motherhood, 107, 119, 161
Motives and motivation, 10, 47, 49, 146, 165, 167
Movies, 137, 145-146, 161, 163. *See also* Films
Multiple drug use, 15-16
Music, 40, 55
Mussen, P., 42
Mythology, 49

Narcotics, 18, 32, 61n, 176, 189
National Clearinghouse for Drug Abuse Information, 46
National Education Association, 33
National Institute on Drug Abuse, 68n, 188
National Merit Scholars, 165
Nature, harmony with, 27-28
Needles, nonsterile, 3
Neighborhoods, factor of, 11, 14-15, 18, 35, 108, 120, 174, 184, 190
Nervous system and neurosis, 125, 145, 173
Nettler, G., 22
New York City, 35, 39, 55
New York State, 14, 21, 36
Newspapers, 48
NIMH supported training center, 34
Nitrous oxide, 71n, 125
Nominees and nominators, 69-70
Nonconformity, 173
Nonprescription drugs, 14, 185
Nonsectarian schools, 183

Nonsmokers, 53, 115
Nonsterile needles, 3
Nonusers of drugs, 47-49, 52, 59
North Allegheny School District, 46
Nowlis, Helen, 39, 189
Nutrition, 41

Obedience, 21, 173
Occupations, factor of, 66, 100, 103, 105, 107, 109
Ohio Department of Education, 46
Opiates, dependency on, 3, 7, 12-13, 31, 60, 83, 110, 187n
Opinion polls, findings of, 18
Overdoses, 3, 18
Over-the-counter drug aids, 2, 15-16, 18

Pain, opiates relief of, 3
Paint thinner, 11, 71n, 125, 127
Parents, 1, 39, 41-44, 55, 64, 123, 133, 138, 172, 183-187; criminal, 56; drug use by, 11; goals of, 140-141; guidance and influence of, 12, 19, 34, 154-155; interviews with, 66, 151; love of, 121; moral support of, 5, 7; morality of, 167; occupations of, 66; permissiveness of, 69, 115-116; supervision by, 13, 16, 119; values of, 27-31, 66; on welfare, 149
Parry, H., 60
Passiveness, 43, 139, 141
Payne, J., 32
Peers: activities, 116-117, approval by, 17-18, 174; group role, 5, 35-46, 106; influence of, 20, 28, 55, 70, 96, 120-121, 135, 138, 186, 190; relationships, 10-13, 66, 100, 107-110; ridicule by, 172-173
Penalties, 25
Pennsylvania, 48, 61
Per capita consumption, 2, 16
Performance: information, 64; reports, 102; school, 1, 15, 21, 106-111, 120, 185
Permissiveness, fallacy of, 69, 115-116, 144-145, 149, 156, 159

Personal: adjustment, 10, 111, 113, 120; conduct, 45; decisions, 135; evaluation, 110, 166; experience, 169; interests, 106, 120; performance, 114; problems, 21, 39, 131-132; relationships, 43; values, 3, 6, 23
Personality traits, 4-5, 10, 15, 21-22, 34, 39, 42, 47, 54, 60, 106, 108, 113, 120, 143-144, 167, 190
Personnel: health, 1; school, 45, 114, 119, 139, 170, 186; training, 27
Pessimism, 176
Petzel, T.P., 59
Pharmaceutical Manufacturer's Association, 46
Pharmacology, 9, 23, 51, 134-135, 140, 174
Physical distress, 1, 28
Physicians, 13, 29, 48, 162, 189
Physiology and inattentiveness, 164-165
Piaget, Jean, 30, 42
Pichot, P., 39
Pills, consumption of, 77, 82-83, 97, 110, 119, 153, 187
Piniuk, J.J., 54
Pleasure seeking, 3, 13, 17-18, 22, 34, 37, 39, 162
Pluralism, 152
Poliakoff, M., 34
Police: careers, 116, 185; juvenile bureau, 189; narcotics department, 18, 176, 189; records, 147; surveillance, 176; youth relationships, 40-41
Policy makers, educational, 6
Political: groups, 184, 189; economic forces, 2; ideologies, 17, 176; themes, 6
Polydrug use, 15
Population, school, 12, 86, 94, 97, 101, 183-184, 186
Portuguese inheritance, 147
"Pot," smoking of, 159
Powders, use of, 110, 187
Pregnancy and drug use, 95
Prescription drugs, 11-12, 60

Prevalence ratio of drugs and users, 70-71, 78, 80, 82, 125, 128
Preventive drug abuse, 2, 5, 7-8, 25, 28, 31-32, 41, 52-55, 82, 85, 132, 174
Primary schools, 43
Principals and vice principals, observations of, 144, 148, 166
Probation authorities, 188
Process education, 36-38, 67, 74, 85, 88-94, 98, 134-137, 165, 170
Professionals and professionalism, 3, 14, 31, 41, 55, 113, 141, 186
Propriety, view of, 2
Prostitution, 14
Psychedelic drugs, 80
Psychiatry, 35, 39, 49, 98, 189
Psychoactive substances, 1-4, 6-16, 21-22, 30, 37, 49, 60, 63, 71, 83, 85, 91, 116, 124, 129-131, 175, 185
Psychoanalysis, 37
Psychology and psychologists, 9-10, 39-40, 49, 52, 66, 174, 184, 189
Psychopathology, 3, 11, 15
Psychopharmacology, 175, 189
Psychotherapy and psychosis, 17, 30, 166
Public Health Service, 95
Punishment and punitive sanctions, 28, 176
Pushers, 153

Questionnaires, 54, 58-59, 65, 69, 74-75, 121, 133, 136, 139-140

Racial situations, 15, 147, 149, 170
Rap sessions, 35
Rape, 29, 185
Rationality, 37, 190
Reading levels, 133
Reason and reality, voice of, 18, 156
Rebelliousness, 19, 22, 145, 157, 174, 176-177
Records: official, 26; police, 147; school, 66, 106, 108, 113, 118, 122, 131; traffic obedience, 116

Recreation, 4, 11-12, 35, 40, 55, 145, 149, 175
Referral channels and programs, 8, 36, 40, 45, 100, 104-109, 112-113, 121, 184
Reform: radical, 46; school, 35, 188; social, 4, 50
Reliability analysis, 42, 50, 59-60, 67-70, 76, 121, 127
Religion, factor of, 3, 11-12, 17-19, 27, 30, 34, 116, 121, 184, 189
Report card history, 100-110, 121
Repression, avoidance of, 27
Research and researchers, 41, 46, 48, 50, 52, 60, 65, 67, 74-76, 95, 136, 139, 175, 188
Resources: community, 45, 188; financial, 39, 41; social, 44
Respiratory infections, 31
Restlessness, element of, 47
Restraints, 13, 138, 190
Risks, levels of, 26, 83
Robins, L.N., 22-23, 56
Roizen, R., 58
Roser, M., 56
Rousseau, Jean Jacques, 27, 35
Rubin, S., 56
Rural areas, 14

Sabotage, 145
Safety, matters of, 2
Salaries, teacher, 2
San Francisco Bay Area, 14, 35
San Mateo County, California, 30, 74
Sanctioned substances, 71-72, 78, 82-84, 101, 106, 110-112, 118, 120, 127-129, 188
Schaps, E., 48-49
Schmidt, W., 59
School: characteristics, 6, 8, 99, 170; nonsectarian, 183; overhead, 2; performance, 1, 15, 21-22, 106-111, 120, 185; personnel, 1, 37, 45, 114, 119, 139, 170, 186; population, 12, 83, 86, 94, 184, 186; records, 66, 106, 108, 113, 118, 122, 131; reform, 35, 188; students, 86,

97, 100-101; training, 20
Schwartz, D.J., 34, 36
Schwilk, G.L., 42
Science and scientific data, 3, 23, 26, 46, 48, 120, 157, 165, 176, 189
Secondary schools, 43, 54
Sedatives, 2-3, 60, 115
Segal, Mark, 34
Self-administered use, 1-2, 129
Self-awareness, 40
Self-concept, 40
Self-confident, 153
Self-control, 13, 27, 37
Self-destructive, 55
Self-discipline, 17-18, 22, 24, 43n
Self-esteem, 34-35, 39, 45, 47
Self-expression, 173
Self-indulgent, 22, 50, 172, 175, 177
Self-injection, 29
Self-medication, 4, 18
Self-realization, 19
Self-referrals, 55
Self-reliance, 159, 172
Self-reports, 61, 63, 67-70, 75-76, 125, 143
Self-restraint, 58
Sensitivity and sensory processes, 2, 163, 165
Separation, marital, 116, 149
Service agencies, 112-113, 121
Sex: factor of, 14, 30, 36, 49, 60, 100; related problems, 102-106
Sexuality, 18, 21
Shoplifting, 14
Shyness, 166, 172
Sleep and sleeping aids, 2, 6, 15, 119, 122, 146, 184
Slimmon, Lee, 34, 36, 54
Smart, R.G., 47-49, 52, 57, 59
Smith, Gene M., 19, 21
Smoking, cigarettes and cannabis, 28, 41, 53, 57-58, 70, 82, 95, 119, 153, 155, 159, 185
Sniffing compounds, 71n, 131
Social: behavior, 5-6, 9-10, 184-186; classes, 14, 16; conduct, 27, 156, 172; experience, 138, 141; forces,

21-23, 113, 152, 175; groups, 11, 13; learning, 29-30, 172-173, 177; life, 3, 136; policies, 16, 24-25, 37; problems, 120, 131-132; reform, 4, 50; relations, 108, 113; resources, 28, 44, 51n, 55, 83, 110, 122; science and scientists, 1, 76, 143-144; studies, 41, 146; workers, 165, 189
Society, 2, 7, 9, 121, 189; forces in, 174; and the law, 28; oppressive, 27
Socioeconomic levels, 5, 14, 19, 43n, 94, 106-107, 112, 119, 149, 165
Sociology, 7, 9, 14, 56
Sociometric study, 75-76
Sociopolitical institutions, 4, 122
Spanish speaking peoples, 14, 110, 121, 146-147
SPARK program, 39, 45, 55-56
Spirits, 71-72
Stamford (Conn.) Curriculum Guide, 46
Stanford Drug Education Project, 8, 138-139, 146, 187-188
Stability: interim, 85, 87-88, 91; maintaining of, 91-92; measuring of, 84-86; overall, 83-85, 88; short-term, 85, 88; and spread, 89-91, 96, 98
Standards, set of, 50
Statistical data, 99, 115, 130n, 138
Statutory delinquency, 177
Step parents, 115-116
Stevenson, H.W., 47
Stimulants, use of, 2, 15-16, 44, 60, 115
STP, 72
Stuart, R.B., 53
Sub-culture, 5, 40, 190
Sugarman, Barry, 43
Supervision: medical, 13, 15, 17, 125; parental, 13, 16, 119
Survey research workers, 188
Swisher, J.D., 8n, 52, 54
Symbols, 30

Tardiness, 145
Teachers: aims of, 38, 136; censure,

Teachers: censure *(cont.)*
172; conscientiousness, 6, 45; control, 150; cooperation, 148, 171; impact of, 5, 48, 93, 95, 133-134, 167; observations by, 111, 118, 144; ratings by, 105-106, 121-122, 131; salaries, 2; student interaction, 67, 141; training of, 29, 34-35, 39-41, 54-55, 184, 187
Teaching: aids and materials, 26-27, 29, 187; at home, 157; methods of, 1, 10, 36-38, 63, 114, 139; and testing procedures, 84, 87, 97, 99-100
Technical assistance, 41, 157
Techniques used, 29-30
Teenagers, activities of, 11-13, 48, 53, 97, 136
Television, influence of, 48, 53, 161, 163
Tempe, Arizona, 21, 54
Tennat, F.S., Jr., 53
Tensions and terrorism, 6, 47, 176
Tests and testing programs: kinds of, 51, 64, 74, 143; nonparametric, 91; and retests, 71, 75-76; statistical, 99, 115, 130n, 138; teacher, 84, 87, 97, 99-100; visual, 74-81, 127; written, 74-81, 127-128
Texas, 53, 176
Theft, 14, 21, 147, 185
Therapy, 60
Thom, D., 21
Thompson, W.D., 54, 171
Thorndike-Lorge word mastery test, 165
Tobacco, use of, 2, 7-8, 15-16, 23, 31, 53, 61n, 69-72, 75-76, 79, 82-84, 110, 127, 129, 131, 176, 187
Tolerance, 153
Toronto, Canada, 49
Traditionalism, social, 122
Traffickers, 25, 116
Training: centers, 34; character, 42, 167, 177; family, 19; intellectual, 43; leadership, 41; personnel, 27; school, 20, 54; teacher, 29, 34-35, 39-41, 54-55, 184, 186-187
Trances, 157
Tranquilizers, use of, 15-19, 60, 119, 122, 155
Transportation, Department of, 46
Treatment, 2, 19; centers, 55
Tresan, D.I., 35-38
Truancy and truants, 21, 100, 105, 107-109, 164, 170, 173; chronic, 56, 150, 154; officers, 147
Turiel, E., 42

Underdeveloped countries, 94n
Unemployment, 149
United Kingdom, 25-28, 32. *See also* England
Universal Research Systems, 46
Unreliability of school records, 108, 118
Unsanctioned substances, 85, 121-122, 165, 188
"Unstable" years, 190
Upper class, 14, 162, 164
Urban poor, 14, 162
Urinalysis testing, 60

Validity figures, 50-51, 67, 76
Valsalva maneuvers, 30
Values: clarification of, 34, 40, 134, 156, 167, 169, 171, 173; community, 167; cultural, 3, 6; family, 66; life, 10; parental, 19, 27-28, 29, 31, 66; personal, 3, 6, 23, 43; sets and issues of, 2, 66, 115, 135-136, 140
Vandalism, 21, 147, 149, 185
Venality, 18
Venereal disease, 28, 41
Violence, fear of, 43, 144, 149, 184-185; television, 163
Visco, E.P., 45, 55
Visits, home, 55, 143, 146
Vocations and vocational patterns, 28-29, 34, 44, 163-164

Warner, R.W., 52
Watson Elementary School, 144, 148-149, 152

Wechsler, H., 21
Weil, A.T., 30-31, 36
Welfare, recipients of, 43, 149, 164
Wetbacks, influx of, 164
Whitehead, P.C., 59
Whitten, P., 42
Wine, use of, 3, 11-12, 18, 31, 71-72, 154, 159
Withdrawal symptoms, 6, 11, 17
Woodcock, J., 25, 33
Work and workers, 121, 162, 165, 188-189

Working class, 14, 39, 149, 162, 164
Workshops, 40, 55, 119
Work-study programs, 28-29
World Health Organization (WHO), 26, 35, 54, 150

Yolles, S.F., 34

Zajonc, R., 53
Zander, G., 49
Zinberg, N.E., 37-38, 45, 49, 172, 174

About the Authors

Richard H. Blum is Director of the Program in Drugs, Crime and Community Studies, Stanford Law School, Stanford University and Chairman of the International Research Group on Drug Legislation and Programs, Geneva, Switzerland. He has served as U.S. Delegate to the United Nations Narcotics Commission and as consultant to the National Institute for Drug Abuse, National Institute of Mental Health, Food and Drug Administration, and the Bureau of Narcotics and Dangerous Drugs. The author of eight books in the drug field, Dr. Blum received the Pacesetter Award from the National Coordinating Council on Drug Education for his research on family life in relationship to drug abuse. With educational experience as a professor of psychology as well as lecturer in psychiatry, criminology and related fields, he served as a founding member of the National Education Association, AANPER, NSTA, NIMH Drug Abuse Education Program. His work, on drug abuse, ranging from epidemiology and psychopharmacology to public policy is internationally known and respected. *Drug Education: Results and Recommendations* is the result of his most recent five-year research and educational activities.

Eva Blum has served as the Co-Director of the Program in Drugs, Crime and Community Studies, Stanford Law School, Stanford University. A child and clinical psychologist, Dr. Blum has been doing research at Stanford on children, young people and drugs since 1960. She has co-authored five books in the drug field, including one on the treatment of alcoholism which is the acknowledged standard in the field. Her interests in mental health, child guidance and preventive work through education to prevent drug abuse have led her to be recognized as an authority in the field.

Emily Garfield is a research associate and graduate of Stanford University. She has been associated with the Program in Drugs, Crime and Community Studies since 1965. Her major efforts have been directed to activities and projects specifically investigating the nonmedical use of psychoactive substances. She has acted in the capacity of interviewer, field coordinator, educator, Assistant Project Director, and most recently, Project Director of a NIDA study on drug education.

About the Authors

Richard H. Blum is Director of the Program in Drugs, Crime and Community Studies, Stanford Law School, Stanford University and Chairman of the International Research Group on Drug Legislation and Programs, Geneva, Switzerland. He has served as U.S. Delegate to the United Nations Narcotics Commission and as consultant to the National Institute for Drug Abuse, National Institute of Mental Health, Food and Drug Administration, and the Bureau of Narcotics and Dangerous Drugs. The author of eight books in the drug field, Dr. Blum received the Pacesetter Award from the National Coordinating Council on Drug Education for his research on family life in relationship to drug abuse. With educational experience as a professor of psychology as well as lecturer in psychiatry, criminology and related fields, he served as a founding member of the National Education Association, AANPER, NSTA, NIMH Drug Abuse Education Program. His work, on drug abuse, ranging from epidemiology and psychopharmacology to public policy is internationally known and respected. *Drug Education: Results and Recommendations* is the result of his most recent five-year research and educational activities.

Eva Blum has served as the Co-Director of the Program in Drugs, Crime and Community Studies, Stanford Law School, Stanford University. A child and clinical psychologist, Dr. Blum has been doing research at Stanford on children, young people and drugs since 1960. She has co-authored five books in the drug field, including one on the treatment of alcoholism which is the acknowledged standard in the field. Her interests in mental health, child guidance and preventive work through education to prevent drug abuse have led her to be recognized as an authority in the field.

Emily Garfield is a research associate and graduate of Stanford University. She has been associated with the Program in Drugs, Crime and Community Studies since 1965. Her major efforts have been directed to activities and projects specifically investigating the nonmedical use of psychoactive substances. She has acted in the capacity of interviewer, field coordinator, educator, Assistant Project Director, and most recently, Project Director of a NIDA study on drug education.